Horses and Money

How to Manage an Equine Business

Also from Blackwell Science

Horse Business Management
Second Edition
Jeremy Houghton Brown and
Vincent Powell-Smith
0 632 03821 7

Keeping Horses
The Working Owner's Guide to
Saving Time and Money
Second Edition
Susan McBane
0 632 03443 2

Horse and Stable Management
Second Edition
Jeremy Houghton Brown and
Vincent Powell-Smith
0 632 03594 3

Horse Care
Jeremy Houghton Brown and
Sarah Pilliner
0 632 03551 X

Getting Horses Fit
A Guide to
Improving Performance
Second Edition
Sarah Pilliner
0 632 03476 9

Horse Nutrition and Feeding
Sarah Pilliner
0 632 03239 1

Equine Science, Health and Performance
Sarah Pilliner and Zoe Davies
0 632 03913 2

Breeding the Competition Horse
Second Edition
John Rose and Sarah Pilliner
0 632 03727 X

Coaching the Rider
Jane Houghton Brown
0 632 03931 0

Teaching Jumping
Jane Houghton Brown
0 632 04127 7

Equine Injury, Therapy and
Rehabilitation
Second Edition
Mary Bromiley
0 632 03608 7

Natural Methods for Equine Health
Mary Bromiley
0 632 03818 7

The Competition Horse
Breeding, Production and
Management
Susan McBane and Gillian McCarthy
0 632 02327 9

Veterinary Manual for the
Performance Horse
N. S. Loving and A. M. Johnston
0 632 03914 0

Horses and Money

How to Manage an Equine Business

Richard Bacon

**Blackwell
Science**

© 1996 by
Blackwell Science Ltd
Editorial Offices:
Osney Mead, Oxford OX2 0EL
25 John Street, London WC1N 2BL
23 Ainslie Place, Edinburgh EH3 6AJ
238 Main Street, Cambridge
  Massachusetts 02142, USA
54 University Street, Carlton
  Victoria 3053, Australia

Other Editorial Offices:
Arnette Blackwell SA
  224, Boulevard Saint Germain
  75007 Paris, France

Blackwell Wissenschafts-Verlag GmbH
  Kurfürstendamm 57
  10707 Berlin, Germany

  Zehetnergasse 6
  A-1140 Wein
  Austria

First published 1996

Set in 10 on 12pt Palatino
by Avocet Typeset, Brill, Aylesbury, Bucks
Printed and bound in Great Britain by
Hartnolls Ltd., Bodmin, Cornwall

The Blackwell Science logo is a
trade mark of Blackwell Science Ltd,
registered at the United Kingdom
Trade Marks Registry

DISTRIBUTORS

Marston Book Services Ltd
PO Box 269
Abingdon
Oxon OX14 4YN
(*Orders:* Tel: 01235 465500
         Fax: 01235 465555)

USA
Blackwell Science, Inc.
238 Main Street
Cambridge, MA 02142
(*Orders:* Tel: 800 215-1000
         617 876-7000
         Fax: 617 492-5263)

Canada
Copp Clark, Ltd
2775 Matheson Blvd East
Mississauga, Ontario
Canada, L4W 4P7
(*Orders:* Tel: 800 263-4374
         905 238-6074)

Australia
Blackwell Science Pty Ltd
54 University Street
Carlton, Victoria 3053
(*Orders:* Tel: 03 9347 0300
         Fax: 03 9349 3016)

A catalogue record for this title
is available from the British Library

ISBN 0–632–04021–1

Library of Congress
Cataloging-in-Publication-Data
Bacon, Richard.
    Horses and money: how to manage
an equine business / by Richard Bacon
      p.   cm.
    Includes index.
    ISBN 0–632–04021–1 (pbk. : alk.
paper)
    1. Horses industry—Management.
HD9434.A2B33   1966
636.1'0068—dc20
                              96–17684
                                   CIP

Contents

Acknowledgements

Thanks are due to a number of people for their help in the completion of this book: my students at Warwickshire College, past and present, whose persistent requests for a suitable text inspired me to start writing; Mr Keith Beaven *BHSI* for his practical comments on my original manuscript, based on years of experience from running a successful business; colleagues at Warwickshire College, especially Jeremy Houghton Brown *BHSSM* (author of the companion volume *Horse Business Management*), Sharon Burt *BHSI* and Philippa Frances *BHSI*.

Introduction

Business Opportunities in the Horse Industry

Horse pursuits are now more popular than they have ever been, with an increasing number of people becoming involved. To match this interest, a significant number of new stables businesses have been set up. In addition, it is the dream of many young people entering the horse industry, through college or traditional training routes, to one day have a yard of their own.

A number of well known businesses have been successful over many years. The reality, however, is that success does not usually come easily in the horse industry, and many businesses last no more than a few years.

Making a success of a business requires a number of factors:

❑   The right business idea – a service that people will want to pay enough money for, and that is marketed effectively.
❑   The right location – a yard with the appropriate facilities; a trekking centre where there is plenty of scenic hacking; a riding school near to a large population.
❑   The right person, with dedication, commitment and a desire to succeed – hallmarks of the horse industry. But in addition they need
❑   The right skills – with horses, people, and the business.

The business skills are often a weakness. It is these that this book addresses, especially the principles of how to manage business finance. Successful yards show that horses and money can go together – this book demonstrates how!

The Role of Financial Management

Every horse business needs money to pay the wages and other expenses. With no money the business will fail. In a thriving yard it is the business that provides the money for its own future and growth. A wealthy minority may be able to inject personal finance to keep a struggling enterprise afloat, but for most people the business must be self-financing. More than this, it should also provide the owner with a reasonable living.

As an introduction, the role of managing business finance can be examined under two headings: the legal requirement and the need for management information.

Legal requirement

All businesses need to keep accurate records of their financial transactions. This is so that:

- ❏ accounts can be prepared for tax assessment at the end of each year
- ❏ Value Added Tax (VAT) returns can be completed periodically. (Calculations in the book are based on the rate of VAT in force at the time of writing, i.e. 17.5%.)

Source documents, such as invoices, and other records need to be carefully filed and stored for several years. This is because they are from time to time inspected by the tax authorities.

Management information

Sound financial management involves much more than meeting the standards of the basic legal requirements. It also needs to provide the information needed to run an efficient business. The manager should consider three different time periods:

- ❏ what has happened in the past
- ❏ the present position
- ❏ future prospects.

The book is divided into three parts to cover these different aspects. Each is supported by examples and illustrations, and a case study which follows the progress of a new yard. Exercises are also included (with answers at the back) to allow practice of the techniques.

The present

This is concerned with keeping on top of the day-to-day issues of invoicing customers, banking receipts, and keeping the records up-to-date. The system should provide enough information to run the business efficiently, and satisfy the legal authorities. This is dealt with in Part 1, What's Going On?

Another aspect is that of monitoring the progress of the business, and controlling it, so that it stays on the right track. Chapter 12, Controlling our Destiny, outlines these principles of 'budgetary control', which help the manager guide the business on a course for success.

The future

The manager of an existing or proposed business needs to know where it is heading. Lenders of finance will want some assurance of this before parting with their depositors' money. The techniques of planning and budgeting, which enable the likely position of the business in the next year or two to be calculated, are discussed in Part 2, Ours is the Future.

The past

How is the business performing? What are its strengths and weaknesses? Looking at past performance may help to find a better way forward for the future. This could be by developing strong points, learning from mistakes, or seeing how weaknesses can be overcome. Part 3, Looking Back – What Happened? shows the different techniques that can be used.

The careful management of past, present and future, taken together, means that the business knows where it is now, where it is going, and has a good chance of getting there. It also avoids falling foul of the tax authorities. The alternative is a disordered situation in the present, failure to learn the lessons of the past, and no future goals to aim for or clear pathway leading to them. In short, sound financial management will mean an improved chance of business success: less likelihood of joining the ranks of former horse business owners.

Part 1
What's Going On?
Essential Records and Accounts

Chapter 1
Where Does the Money Come From?
Sources of Finance

It has already been noted that every business needs money. The funds required to start and continue an enterprise can come from a number of sources, such as the owner, or borrowing in different forms. These are summarised in Figure 1.1.

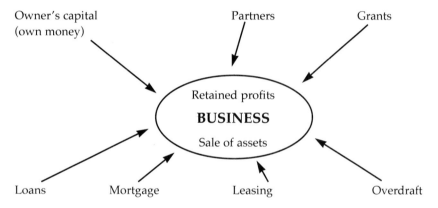

Figure 1.1   Sources of business finance

Internal Sources

An internal source of finance is money that comes from within the business, rather than from some outside body such as a lender or the business owner.

Retained profits

This is the money made by the business activities, which can then be used to:

❑ pay the day-to-day expenses such as feed and wages
❑ reduce borrowing, *or*
❑ reinvest in the holding.

It is vital that the business generates sufficient cash in this way. If it does not:

❑ debts to lenders may increase

❑   the business could become run down through lack of investment.

In the end these will both lead to business failure – unless the owner can keep pumping money in to keep it afloat.

Sale of business assets

Sometimes it may be sensible to sell an asset to provide funds for a more useful one. For example, an outlying field unsuitable for grazing may be sold to pay for an indoor school. If such an action is forced by financial pressures and the need to repay debts, then it shows that the business is in a seriously poor state of health.

Owner's Capital

The amount of money invested in a business by the owner must be a sufficiently high proportion of the total funding. If it is not, the level of borrowing will be too great for the business to be able to pay the interest charges and make the repayments when they become due.

Anyone thinking of starting up in business should seriously consider whether they have enough of their own money behind them. If they have not, they will find it difficult to borrow further sums of money from commercial lenders, and their chances of success are slim.

Money from family, friends, or partners in the business venture can also be included in this category, if it is offered as a gift rather than as a loan.

Grants

A large number of grants and government or charitable schemes are available, some of which may be able to offer financial help to the new or developing horse business. It is impossible to list them in a book of this nature, because many are limited in their availability and the situation is constantly changing. Some banks offer a grants advisory service where, for a fee, a search can be made for any schemes that may be able to help a particular project. Other possible sources of advice are:

❑   the Agricultural Development and Advisory Service (ADAS)
❑   Rural Development Commission
❑   the local Training and Enterprise Council (TEC)

Specific sources of assistance worthy of mention are given here.

Farm diversification grants

For several years the Ministry of Agriculture, Fisheries and Food (MAFF) has been offering farm diversification grants to farmers wishing to develop alternative sources of income. Some horse enterprises have been eligible for aid. These grants have been available only to full time farmers, and have covered feasibility studies and marketing as well as capital investments. Details of the current situation can be obtained from offices of the MAFF.

Enterprise Allowance Scheme

This provides help to people starting their own business by paying a regular income for the first year. It is restricted to people who have been registered as unemployed prior to starting their business. The latest details are available from the local Training and Enterprise Council (TEC).

The Prince's Trust

The Prince's Trust (until early 1996 called the Prince's Youth Business Trust) can help young people between the ages of 18 and 29 to get started in business. A contact number can be found in local telephone directories.

Borrowing

Almost all businesses use some form of borrowing, and this is likely to be a very important source of finance to a new venture. Different types of borrowing are suitable for distinct purposes, and can be considered under headings of short-, medium- and long-term. These are shown in Table 1.1.

Table 1.1   Sources of borrowing

	Short-term	**Medium-term**	**Long-term**
Years	Up to 1	2–5	Up to 25
Purposes	Day-to-day expenses such as feed and wages	Machinery, vehicles, school horses, breeding stock	Property, buildings, arenas, land
Forms	Overdraft Trade credit	Loans Hire purchase Leasing	Loans Mortgage

Overdraft

The main features of a bank overdraft are:

❑   It is a facility to overdraw the current account, up to a limit which needs to be agreed in advance.

❏   The limit will be reviewed by the bank manager at least once a year.
❏   Interest is only charged on the amount that the account is overdrawn, making an overdraft the most flexible, and often cheapest, form of borrowing.
❏   The bank manager can ask for it to be repaid at short notice.

The rate of interest charged will be the Bank of England base rate plus somewhere between 2.5% and 6%, depending on the circumstances of the borrower. Major influences will be their track record, and the financial security of the business.

It is unwise to use an overdraft for long-term investments, but rather to meet short-term needs for extra cash. An example would be to buy a horse which will be kept for a few weeks before being sold at a profit, thus enabling the overdraft to be repaid.

Trade credit

This is the time that is allowed by suppliers between a business receiving goods and paying for them. The length of time given depends on the relationship between the purchaser and supplier. Trade credit is a common arrangement between businesses, but not one that should be abused by extending the credit period beyond what was agreed. Such an action can very quickly gain a business a reputation of being a poor payer. Even taking the full period of credit allowed can sometimes cost a business money through the loss of early payment discounts.

Business loans

A loan differs from an overdraft in a number of ways:

❏   It is a set sum of money, usually borrowed for a specific purpose.
❏   The amount can be for sums of £1,000 upwards.
❏   It is repayable over an agreed period ranging from 1 year up to 25 years.
❏   A fixed schedule to repay the money borrowed, plus interest, will be part of the agreement.
❏   The lender cannot demand early repayment unless instalments have not been paid when they were due.

A loan should not be taken out for a longer period than the expected life of the asset it is being used to obtain. For a vehicle this would usually mean a maximum of five years. The size of loan repayments can be worked out using the *amortisation table* (Table 1.2).

Example: to repay a loan of £15,000 over 10 years at 12% interest:
Annual charge per £1,000 = £177
×15 = £2,655 per year

Some form of security is often required for larger loans. This will enable the lender to recover their money in the event of unforeseen circumstances, such as the business failing.

Table 1.2 Amortisation table

Write-off period (years)	Annual charge to write off £1,000						
	Interest rate (%)						
	6	8	10	12	14	16	18
5	237	250	264	277	291	305	320
6	203	216	230	243	257	271	286
7	179	192	205	219	233	248	262
8	161	174	187	201	216	230	245
9	147	160	174	188	202	217	232
10	136	149	163	177	192	207	223
15	103	117	131	147	163	179	196
20	87	102	117	134	151	169	187
25	78	94	110	127	145	164	183

Commercial mortgage

A commercial mortgage is a loan especially for the purchase of business premises. The mortgage is a legal document, securing the loan to the deeds of the property so that the lender can sell the premises to recoup their money, if the need arises. The amount of the loan will usually be restricted to 80% of the premises valuation, and will often be repayable over 25 years.

There are two common ways to repay a mortgage:

❑ The annuity method – regular repayments are made which consist of interest and part of the sum borrowed. At the end of the term of the mortgage, the total sum has been repaid.
❑ The endowment method of repayment is linked to a life assurance (endowment) policy, to which regular premiums are paid. Only interest is paid to the lender until the term of the mortgage is completed. At this point the endowment policy matures, providing the money to repay the borrowing.

Hire purchase

Machinery and vehicles are frequently bought by hire purchase. When receiving the item, a deposit has to be paid. This is followed by regular instalments over an agreed period to a finance company. These cover the remainder of the cost, plus interest. The buyer only becomes the legal owner when the final instalment has been made. Early repayment of a hire purchase agreement can be very expensive.

Leasing

Leasing is another form of funding offered by finance companies. They buy the asset, for example a vehicle, and give it to the lessee in return for rental payments over the period of the lease. It is a common way for businesses to acquire vehicles, machinery and office equipment like computers and photocopiers. A number of variations are possible with leasing agreements, such as ownership transferring to the lessee at the end of the period, or the inclusion of maintenance within the lease.

Comparing sources of borrowing

Several factors may need to be considered, such as the costs incurred to arrange the borrowing, or the flexibility of the agreement. A major consideration will be the rate of interest charged. This is best assessed by looking at the annual percentage rate, or APR. It is the most accurate measure of what it will cost to borrow money, and is defined as:

'The annual cost, in interest and fees, expressed as a percentage of the sum borrowed.'

Lenders are required by law to state the APR that will be charged.

What the lender is looking for

A range of factors will be carefully considered before the lender agrees to lend the money.

Integrity

The track record of the borrower in repaying debts; whether they have consistently honoured agreements, or have become credit 'blacklisted'. The ability and experience of the borrower will also be important.

Purpose

Whether the money is required for a sensible business reason which is likely to make a worthwhile return.

Amount

The sum of money requested, and whether this will actually be sufficient for the purpose.

Repayments

The lender will require the money to be repaid in regular instalments, and must be satisfied that the proposals will enable this. They will also consider here whether the business will become over-borrowed.

Term

How long the money will be borrowed for. This should be matched to the purpose of the loan. Making repayments over a longer term costs less on a monthly or annual basis, but is more expensive in the long run.

Security

In case of problems that prevent the borrowing from being repaid as planned, the lender may want some form of security which will enable the money to be recovered. This could take the form of:

- ❏ title deeds to property
- ❏ life assurance policies that have acquired a surrender value
- ❏ stocks and shares
- ❏ someone who is prepared to guarantee the loan.

When considering different sources of funding, especially for a large investment, it is best to look at what is being offered by various lenders. The advice of an accountant can often be helpful to consider the overall implications for the business, and any taxation issues that might be involved.

Sale of Shares

The sale of shares is an option that is not available to all businesses, but only to those that are operating as a limited company. The most common forms of business, which are the sole trader and the partnership, are unable to sell shares.

Private limited company status may be worth considering, not just for the ability to raise money by selling shares. Another factor is that the liability of the owners for the debts of the company is limited to their investment in it, whereas a sole trader or partner can lose all of their money.

There are various other arguments for and against becoming incorporated, and it is best to seek professional advice which can allow for individual circumstances.

Chapter 2
Controlling Paperwork
Business Documents and Office Organisation

The starting point for effective management of money is a good record keeping system. This needs to include book-keeping for financial transactions, and also enterprise records for specific activities of the business.

Enterprise Records

The types of records needed will depend on the activities of the business, but some examples are:

❏ Livery record – showing the contracted livery fee, and any extra services that have been provided and which will be charged to the client.
❏ Riding school – an individual record for each horse, which will show how much work they do. This will show up any horses or ponies that are less popular or tend to need time off. It could also include veterinary and farrier expenses.
❏ Stud record – similar to that for a livery record, needed to keep account of all the costs for each visiting mare. Another record needs to be kept for stallions to show how many mares they have received.

Book-keeping

A book-keeping system needs to satisfy a number of different criteria:

❏ the legal requirement to keep records up to the standard demanded for Value Added Tax (VAT) and income tax purposes;
❏ the information needed to manage the business efficiently, by giving answers to questions such as:
How much has been spent, and on what?
What income has been received?
Who is owed money, and what debts are owed to the business?
What is the bank balance?
Is the business making any money?

For a book-keeping system to satisfy all of these criteria, an organised system for handling and recording the paperwork that is involved with buying and selling is needed.

Purchases

A typical purchasing transaction is likely to involve the exchange of a number of documents. The most important are summarised in Figure 2.1.

Buyer	Document	Supplier
	<— Catalogue/ price list ———	Details of products
Order placed ——	Purchase order ———>	
	<— Delivery note ———	Goods delivered
	<— Invoice ———	Request for payment
	<— Statement ———	Summary of payments and invoices
Payment made ——	Cheque and remittance advice ———>	

Figure 2.1 Purchase documents

Orders

A large organisation will insist that orders are always made in writing, using the company's official order form. This is so that a record is available to show what has been ordered and by whom. In the smaller business the order is often verbal, given over the telephone or directly to the salesperson, but the use of a written order form is still advisable. It provides hard evidence of what has actually been ordered, in case of mistakes or disputes occurring. Printed order forms, or simply a duplicate book, can be used.

The details on the order should be as precise as possible, with the price taken from the supplier's catalogue or from a verbal enquiry. A signature is vital to give authorisation to the order. The second copy should be filed in an order file, or left in the order duplicate book, until the goods have been received.

An example of a written order is shown in Figure 2.2.

Delivery note

This is sent by the supplier along with the goods. The person receiving the delivery needs to check that:

❑ everything is present and in good condition
❑ the delivery corresponds with the order.

The delivery note can then be signed and dated. If it is not possible to check the delivery, the words 'Contents not inspected' should be written on it. An example delivery note is shown in Figure 2.3.

PURCHASE ORDER
OXHILL STABLES
Oxhill Farm
Nether Compton
Midshire
NC10 4TF
(01623) 123456

To: **Order No: 103**

Feed Supplies Ltd
Valley Road Ind.Estate
Windmarsh
Midshire
NC14 7PQ

Date: 12 September 199_

Ref.	Quantity	Description	Unit Price £
HOR01	12 bags	Horse & Pony Nuts, 25 kg bags	6.00
COO01	6 bags	Cool Mix, 20 kg bags	5.20
SBP01	4 bags	Sugar Beet Pulp Nuts, 25 kg bags	3.00

Signed: *L J Clark*   **Date:** *12/9/199_*

Figure 2.2   Purchase order

Invoice

This is the most important document, which must be filed away safely. The Inland Revenue require that invoices are kept for seven years in case of income tax inspections. They are also important as evidence that the business has paid money, and so will need to be seen by the accountant.

An invoice must contain a number of details to come up to the standard required for Value Added Tax. These are illustrated on the invoice in Figure 2.4.

Important points that must be included are:

❑ Date/tax point – this is the transaction date for VAT purposes, and is usually the same as the invoice date, unless the issue of the invoice has been delayed.
❑ VAT registration number.
❑ Invoice number.
❑ Quantity, description and unit price – must be stated for each item.
❑ Total goods – the value of goods or services before VAT has been added.
❑ VAT – the rate and amount of Value Added Tax.

DELIVERY NOTE
Feed Supplies Ltd
Valley Road Industrial Estate
Windmarsh
Midshire
NC14 7PQ
Tel.(01623) 987665

Deliver To: **Delivery Note No:** 14133

> Miss L Clark
> Oxhill Stables
> Oxhill Farm
> Nether Compton
> Midshire
> NC10 4TF

Date: 14/09/199_   **Your Order No:** 103
Account No: CLAR01

Ref.	Quantity	Description
HOR01	12 bags	Horse & Pony Nuts, 25 kg bags
COO01	6 bags	Cool Mix, 20 kg bags
SBP01	4 bags	Sugar Beet Pulp Nuts, 25 kg bags

Received:
Signed: *L J Clark*   **Name:** *LINDA CLARK*
Date: 14/9/199_

Figure 2.3   Delivery note

❑   Amount due – the total value of the invoice.
❑   Terms – such as when payment must be made, or any discount terms offered. The letters E&OE are sometimes printed, which stand for Errors and Omissions Excepted. This gives the supplier the right to change the invoice if a mistake is discovered.

On receipt of an invoice, it should be checked against the order and delivery note. If there are any errors or discrepancies, it should be returned with a query to the supplier.

Credit note

A credit note is given instead of making a refund if:

❑   there has been a mistake on an invoice
❑   goods have been returned.

INVOICE
Feed Supplies Ltd
Valley Road Industrial Estate
Windmarsh
Midshire
NC14 7PQ
Tel (01623) 987665
VAT registration no: 322 5524 76

To: **Invoice No:** 12193

Miss L Clark
Oxhill Stables
Oxhill
Nether Compton
Midshire
NC10 4TF

Date/Tax Point: 16/09/199_   **Your Order No:** 103
Account No: CLAR01

Ref.	Quantity	Description	VAT rate %	Price £ /unit	Total £
HOR01	12 bags	Horse & Pony Nuts, 25 kg bags	0	6.00	72.00
COO01	6 bags	Cool Mix, 20 kg bags	0	5.20	31.20
SBP01	4 bags	Sugar Beet Pulp nuts, 25 kg bags	0	3.00	12.00
		Goods total			115.20
		VAT @ 17.5%			0.00
		Total amount due			115.20

Terms: Net 14 days

Figure 2.4   Invoice

The value of the credit note can then be offset against any invoices the next time that the supplier is paid. The layout and contents are very similar to those of an invoice, and are illustrated in Figure 2.5. The credit note will usually state the reason for credit at the bottom.

Statement of account

Regular suppliers will issue a statement each month, to summarise transactions that have occurred during the period, and show any outstanding balance, as illustrated in Figure 2.6.

CREDIT NOTE
Feed Supplies Ltd
Valley Road Industrial Estate
Windmarsh
Midshire
NC14 7PQ
Tel (01623) 987665
VAT registration no: 322 5524 76

To: **Credit Note No:**   5422

Miss L Clark
Oxhill Stables
Oxhill
Nether Compton
Midshire
NC10 4TF

Date/Tax Point: 19/09/199_   **Invoice No:**   12193
Account No: CLAR01   **Your Order No:** 103

Ref.	Quantity	Description	VAT rate %	Price £ /unit	Total £
HOR01	2 bags	Horse & Pony Nuts, 25 kg bags	0	6.00	12.00
		Goods Total			12.00
		VAT @ 17.5%			0.00
		Total amount			12.00

Reason for credit:
Goods returned damaged

Figure 2.5   Credit note

Remittance advice

A remittance advice is usually included with an invoice or statement. It is returned to the supplier when making payment, and will show the invoices that are being paid. Thus it helps the accounts department of the supplier to relate cheques received to the invoices that are being paid.

Controlling the paperwork

With so many documents involved, an organised system for handling them is needed. An effective one for the small business is to have a stack of three filing trays, labelled:

❏   Goods inward

STATEMENT
Feed Supplies Ltd
Valley Road Industrial Estate
Windmarsh
Midshire
NC14 7PQ
(01623) 987665
VAT registration no: 322 5524 76

To:

Miss L Clark
Oxhill Stables
Oxhill Farm
Nether Compton
Midshire
NC10 4TF

Date: 30/09/199_   **Account No:** CLAR01

Date	Details	Debit	Credit	Balance
01/09	Balance			155.80
05/09	Payment		155.80	
16/09	Invoice 12193	115.20		
19/09	CN 5422		12.00	
30/09	Due for payment			103.20

Figure 2.6   Statement of account

❑ For payment
❑ Paid

These can store the documents until the regular (weekly or monthly) payment and book-keeping session.

Different documents can be handled in the following way:

❑ Purchase orders – kept in the order file, or order book, until the delivery has been received.
❑ Delivery notes – when the goods have been received, the order is compared to the delivery note. They are then pinned together and stored in the 'Goods Inward' tray.
❑ Invoice – this needs to be checked. If there are no problems, the order

and delivery note can be thrown away. The invoice should then be stored in the 'For payment' tray.

❑ Statements, remittance advices or credit notes should also be stored in the 'For Payment' tray, with documents from the same supplier attached together.

If a large number of invoices are received, it is a good idea to record them in a purchases book (Figure 2.7 is an example of the details to be shown).

Date	Supplier	Invoice number	Invoice total	Goods	VAT	Progress
16/9	Feed supplies	12193	115.20	115.20	0.00	Paid 30/9
21/9	British Telecom	4323523	258.65	220.13	38.52	Paid 30/9

Figure 2.7   Purchases book

Details of payment, or any queries, can be entered in the 'Progress' column. A quick look at the book will show which invoices are unpaid and need to be settled, rather than having to sort through piles of paper.

❑ Receipts for cash payments, or invoices that have been paid, go into the 'Paid' tray.

Making payment

On a regular basis, which can be weekly or monthly, unpaid invoices should be sorted and due accounts paid. An appropriate procedure to follow is outlined below.

(1) Empty the 'For Payment' tray, and sort the invoices into those that should be paid now, and those that can be left for another day. Factors to consider here will be:
   ❑ the date of the invoice and the payment terms
   ❑ loss of early payment discounts
   ❑ the size of the invoice relative to the available money.

(2) Having selected the accounts to be paid, group the invoices (and any credit notes) from the same supplier together. Arrange all documents in alphabetical order.

(3) Write out the cheques, in alphabetical order of suppliers, remembering to complete the cheque book stubs. Make a note of:
   ❑ the invoice number on the back of the cheque
   ❑ the cheque number and payment date on the invoice.
   Fill in any necessary details on remittance advices.

(4) Before posting the cheques, complete the cash analysis book (details of this are given in the next chapter), working from the invoices.

Transactions should be entered in date order, so record any documents in the 'Paid' tray before the invoices that have just been paid.

(5) A useful checking procedure at this point is to compare the details on the cheques with the cash analysis book entries. If any differences are found, a mistake has been made, which can be corrected before the cheques are posted.

(6) Finally, the cheques (plus remittance advices) can be posted. Paid invoices and receipts should be filed away securely in a box file. They should be in cheque number order so that they will be easy to find in the future, should the need arise.

Sales

There are two distinct types of sales:

❏ Credit sales – when the customer is invoiced for goods or services.
❏ Cash sales – payment is made at the time of sale, either by cash or cheque.

Credit sales

For most stables, credit sales will involve the raising of invoices to customers, and receiving payment. At times it may be necessary to issue reminders to late payers. Invoices should be raised promptly, or on a regular basis for on-going services such as livery. Separate records (enterprise records) will usually need to be kept to allow the invoices to be completed accurately.

Any sales invoices issued should be recorded in a sales book, which is similar to the purchases book illustrated above. This will show, at a glance, who has not paid their bill. A copy of the invoice should be kept, which can be stored temporarily in a tray marked 'Sales invoices'.

When payment is received, this should be recorded in the sales book, and the payment date noted on the copy sales invoice (an example is shown in Figure 2.8).

Date	Customer	Invoice number	Invoice total	Goods	VAT	Progress
31/8	P. Tweedie	1221	282.00	240.00	42.00	Paid 8/9
31/8	V. Late	1222	211.50	180.00	31.50	Reminder 21/9
30/9	P. Tweedie	1223	282.00	240.00	42.00	
30/9	T. Jump	1224	235.00	200.00	35.00	

Figure 2.8   Sales book

Cash sales

If there is a significant number of cash sales, an electronic cash till is advisable for efficiency and security reasons. This will provide a printed record of each transaction, as well as daily totals. Where cash sales are less frequent, each transaction should be recorded in a cash book, noting the date, name of payee, amount and receipt number. At the end of each day the total receipts should be calculated and checked against the takings in the cash box.

Banking receipts

Money received should be kept securely until it can be banked. Procedures to follow include:

- ❏ Make sure that the date, amount (in words and figures), payee's name and signature, are all correct and present on cheques.
- ❏ Details of cash and cheques to be banked have to be entered onto the paying-in slip, with every cheque noted on the back of the slip and the counterfoil.

Role of computers

An increasing number of businesses now own a computer, which can be put to many uses in the stables office. Accounts programmes can cope with a wide range of financial management functions. These range from the ordering and invoicing procedures described in this chapter, to book-keeping, VAT returns, and preparation of accounts statements. A number of commercial packages are available. More advanced programmes can also incorporate budget targets and monitor the progress of the business against these.

Introducing a computerised system will involve an initial investment of both finance and time, but can reap significant returns through greater efficiency and improved access to data.

Chapter 3
That's the Way the Money Goes
Basic Book-keeping

An effective book-keeping system provides the key to the whole area of managing money and lies at the heart of the accounting process, which is vital for the legal and management reasons given in the previous chapter. The overall process is shown in Figure 3.1.

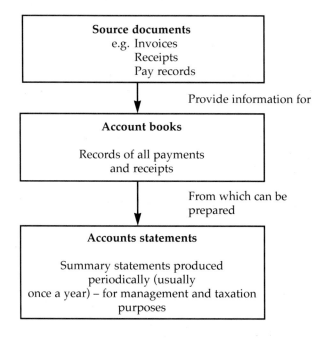

Figure 3.1 The accounting process

Cash Analysis

A system of book-keeping suitable for most horse businesses is cash analysis. The main features of this system are:

❑   an account book is kept for each financial year
❑   receipts and payments are recorded on separate pages

❑   figures are only entered when money has actually been received or paid.

Each transaction is entered on a separate line of the account book. The columns are given various headings, the first three always being:

Date   which is the date of receipt or payment
Detail   the name of the customer or supplier, and what the money is for
Amount   the sum of money exchanged.

The remaining columns are known as analysis columns, and these are used to record different categories of income or payment. For example, appropriate receipts headings may be:

Stud: *Riding school:*
Stud fees   Lessons
Mare's livery   Hacks
Youngstock   Competitions

Completing the cash analysis book

Each transaction is entered twice, first in the amount column, and then in an analysis column. This can be illustrated by an example, for a stud which has received the following:

❑   Mr Smith paid £3,200 for 3-year old Goodnight Boy on 8 June 1996.
❑   Mrs Foale paid £300 on 12 June 1996, for stud fee of £200 and mare's livery of £100.

The cash analysis book entries would be as shown in Figure 3.2.

Date	Detail	Amount	Youngstock	Stud fees	Mare's livery
8/6	Mr Smith – Goodnight Boy	3,200.00	3,200.00		
12/6	Mrs Foale – stud fee and livery for Best Chance	300.00		200.00	100.00
	Total for June	3,500.00	3,200.00	200.00	100.00

Figure 3.2   Cash analysis book entries – receipts

At the end of every month, the book is completed and the total for each column calculated, as shown in Figure 3.2.

To check that the entries are correct, add up the totals of the analysis columns. These should give the same figure as the total in the Amount column. If they do not, a mistake has been made which needs to be corrected. This cross checking is also illustrated in Figure 3.2:

Analysis column totals	£
Youngstock	3,200
Stud fees	200
Mare's livery	100
	3,500 – the same as the Amount column total.

Start a new page for each month. On the top row, enter the totals for each column brought forward from the previous month.

Continuing the example above, if June is the first month of the financial year, the page for July will start by showing the totals brought forward from June. At the end of July, a total will be calculated both for July's transactions, and for a cumulative total for the year to date. This is illustrated in Figure 3.3. In this way, the figures build up for the whole year.

Date	Detail	Amount	Youngstock	Stud fees	Mare's livery
1/7	Total brought forward	3,500	3,200	200	100
	Entries for July	...	...	...	...
	Total for July	5,800	4,000	1,200	600
	Cumulative total	9,300	7,200	1,400	700

Figure 3.3   Cash analysis book – monthly and cumulative totals

Payments are dealt with in the same manner, although more column headings are usually needed, and some items may need to be grouped together. The analysis column headings should be grouped in the following order, to help with preparing accounts at the end of the year:

❑ Direct costs – horses purchased, feed, bedding, veterinary and medicines, farrier costs, etc.
❑ Overheads – labour, rates, vehicle costs, administration, and the other expenses of the business.
❑ Capital investments in buildings, machinery, etc., and loan repayments.
❑ Private - money taken out of the business for personal living expenses, and tax payments.

Value Added Tax (VAT)

This section describes how to include VAT in the book-keeping system. Further details about VAT are given in chapter 21, and it may be helpful to read them before proceeding.

Calculating VAT

It will often be necessary to work out the VAT that is involved in transactions.

(1) VAT to add on to a price.
This is found by the formula:
$$\text{VAT} = \text{price (excluding VAT)} \times \frac{\text{VAT rate \%}}{100}$$
With VAT at 17.5%, the tax to add on to a livery fee of £65 would be:
$$\text{VAT} = £65 \times \frac{17.5}{100} = £11.37$$
Hence total price £76.37.

(2) When the price includes VAT.
A different formula has to be used:
$$\text{VAT} = \frac{\text{Price (including VAT)} \times \text{VAT rate \%}}{(100 + \text{VAT rate})}$$

i.e. if the VAT rate is 17.5%, the formula is:
$$\text{VAT} = \frac{\text{Price (including VAT)} \times 17.5}{117.5}$$

Working backwards from the example above:
$$\text{VAT} = £76.37 \times \frac{17.5}{117.5} = £11.37$$

The VAT is always rounded down to the nearest whole penny. If a discount is offered on a price, the tax is calculated on the discounted figure.

VAT registration

When a business becomes registered for VAT, the book-keeping system needs to be adapted to cope with the tax. The actual records that need to be kept depend on the size of the business. Most horse businesses are small enough to qualify for the Cash Accounting Scheme, which enables records to be kept in the cash analysis book. Always check with an accountant if in doubt about the need to register, or eligibility for the Cash Accounting Scheme.

If keeping records in the cash analysis book, the following columns need to be added:

In receipts:
VAT on sales – to record any VAT received on sales.
Value of sales – showing the value of sales, without VAT.

In payments:
VAT on inputs – for VAT paid on purchases.
VAT to C&E – to record payments of VAT to Customs and Excise, after VAT returns have been completed.

Value of inputs – to record the value of business inputs that need to be included in the VAT return. The main items not included in this column are wages, private drawings and tax, VAT, and finance costs.

Entries in the cash analysis book are the same as before, except that the VAT and the value of the goods or service need to be recorded in separate analysis columns. The value of the goods or service (net of VAT) also needs to be entered in the Value of Inputs or Sales column.

For example, a livery stables has received the following money:

❑   Mr Green – £235, comprising livery fees of £200, plus £35 VAT, on 21 August.
❑   Miss Zaffar – £246.75, comprising livery fees of £180, additional services of £30, plus £36.75 VAT on 27 August.

The cash analysis book entries will be as shown in Figure 3.4.

Date	Detail	Amount	Livery	Other services	VAT on sales	Value of sales
21/8	Mr Green	235.00	200.00		35.00	200.00
27/8	Miss Zaffar	246.75	180.00	30.00	36.75	210.00

Figure 3.4   Cash analysis book entries with VAT

VAT returns

At regular intervals, usually every three months, a VAT return has to be completed. The figures for this can be taken from the cash analysis book totals for the period. To illustrate, the relevant sections of the book for the quarter June to August are shown in Figure 3.5. These figures will be used to complete the VAT return as shown in Figure 3.6.

Receipts

Date	Detail	Amount	...	...	VAT on sales	Value of sales
31/8	Total June–Aug	8,812.50	...	...	1,312.50	7,500.00

Payments

Date	Detail	Amount	...	VAT on inputs	Value of inputs	VAT to C&E
31/8	Total June–Aug	7,400.00	...	632.00	4,250.00	

Figure 3.5   Extracting figures for the VAT return from the cash analysis book

Value Added Tax Return
For the period
01/06/__ to 31/08/__

		£	p
VAT due in this period on *sales* and other outputs	1	1,312	50
VAT due in this period on *acquisitions* from other EC member states	2	None	
Total VAT due (the sum of boxes 1 and 2)	3	1.312	50
VAT reclaimed in this period on *purchases* and other inputs (including acquisitions from the EC)	4	632	00
Net VAT to be paid to Customs or reclaimed by you (*difference* between boxes 3 and 4)	5	680	50
Total value of sales and all other outputs excluding any VAT (include your box 8 figure)	6	7,500	00
Total value of purchases and all other inputs excluding any VAT (include your box 9 figure)	7	4,250	00
Total value of all supplies of goods and related services excluding any VAT to other EC member states	8	None	
Total value of all acquisitions of goods and related services excluding any VAT from other EC member states	9	None	

Figure 3.6   Example VAT return entries

Having made a repayment of VAT, an entry can be made in the VAT to C&E column (Figure 3.7).

Payments

Date	Detail	Amount	...	VAT on inputs	Value of inputs	VAT to C&E
5/9	C&E VAT repayment	680.50	...			680.50

Figure 3.7   Entering a VAT repayment to Customs and Excise

Bank Reconciliation

The bank reconciliation is another checking procedure, which should be carried out every month. It involves comparing the bank statement and cash analysis book to spot any differences. These may be due to:

- ❏   errors (by book-keeper or bank, usually book-keeper)
- ❏   fraud
- ❏   items getting missed such as direct debits or bank interest charges
- ❏   delays in cheques clearing.

Any differences need to be looked into to find out what the correct figure should be.

The procedure is as follows:

(1) Find an entry on the bank statement to correspond with each cash analysis book entry. Tick if correct, and investigate any differences. Payments are usually straightforward, but an important point to remember with receipts is that if a number of items are paid into the bank at the same time, only one entry will appear on the bank statement.

(2) Enter into the cash analysis book any items that have been missed, such as direct debits, bank interest and charges.

(3) Calculate the totals for the month in the cash analysis book.

(4) It is now possible to calculate a projected bank balance. This shows how much money will be in the account after all transactions undertaken have cleared, using the formula:

Closing bank balance for month (from bank statement)
+ Receipts banked but not yet on the statement
– Payments made but not yet on the statement
⎯⎯
= Projected bank balance

For example, the bank statement for October shows a closing bank balance of £4,000. £100 has been paid into the account, but cheques for £2,500 have recently been sent to suppliers. The projected balance is:

	£
Opening bank balance	4,000
Receipts banked	100
Payments made	(2,500)
Projected bank balance	1,600

The actual position of the business is therefore not as good as the bank statement suggests.

Petty Cash

The cash analysis system does not cope very well with small cash purchases, so it is best to use a separate system for these items of 'petty cash'. Book-keeping is made more simple if cash receipts are kept separate from cash payments. The receipts should be banked along with other forms of income, and a petty cash box used to make payments.

A commonly used system for petty cash is the imprest system. Its main features are:

- ❏ A sum of money, or float, is established in the petty cash box every week or month.
- ❏ Only an authorised person is permitted to unlock the box and take money out.
- ❏ Requests for payment should be supported by a receipt.
- ❏ A petty cash voucher is filled out and signed by the person receiving the money.
- ❏ An entry is also made in the petty cash book.
- ❏ A check can be made that the correct money is in the box, at any time, by adding up the total value of vouchers and cash. These should equal the amount of the float.
- ❏ At the end of the period, the petty cash book is totalled and cash withdrawn from the bank to restore the balance in the petty cash box back to the float.

An example of a petty cash book is shown in Figure 3.8.

Receipts	Date	Details	Voucher no.	Total payment	Postage	Stationery	Other	VAT
50.00	1/10	Balance brought forward						
	3/10	Stamps	1	4.20	4.20			
	4/10	Pens, pencils	2	3.30		2.81		0.49
	4/10	Note paper	3	7.50		6.39		1.11
	6/10	Milk	4	2.71			2.71	
	7/10	Coffee and tea	5	4.28			4.28	
				21.99	4.20	9.20	6.99	1.60
21.99	7/10	Cash from bank						
		Balance carried forward		50.00				

Figure 3.8   Oxhill Stables petty cash book

Case Study

This is the first of a number of case study sections concerned with Linda Clark and her business, Oxhill Stables. It is the end of May, and Linda's livery yard and riding school has been running for just over one year. She has established a routine of completing the books at the end of each month, and has produced the information in Figures 3.9 and 3.10 for May.

Date	Detail	Amount	Riding lessons	Livery fees	Sundry income	VAT on sales	Value of sales
01/05	Brought forward	9,341.25	6,100.00	1,650.00	200.00	1,391.25	7,950.00
03/05	L. Platt – livery	311.38		255.00	10.00	46.38	265.00
07/05	Lessons wc 3/5	1,670.00	1,421.28			248.72	1,421.28
08/05	M. Crisp – livery	305.50		260.00		45.50	260.00
12/05	P. Tweedie – livery	90.48		65.00	12.00	13.48	77.00
14/05	Lessons wc 10/5	1,710.00	1,455.32			254.68	1,455.32
21/05	Lessons wc 17/5	1,735.00	1,476.60			258.40	1,476.60
23/05	H. Jump – livery	90.00		76.60		13.40	76.60
26/05	T. Long – livery	450.03		383.00		67.03	383.00
28/05	Lessons wc 24/5	1,695.00	1,442.55			252.45	1,442.55
30/05	V. Late – livery	405.38		320.00	25.00	60.38	345.00
	Total for May	8462.77	5,795.74	1,359.60	47.00	1,260.42	7,202.34
	Cum. total Apr–May	17,804.02	11,895.74	3,009.60	247.00	2,651.67	15,152.34

Figure 3.9   Oxhill Stables – cash analysis book – receipts

Date	Detail	Ch.	Amount	Feed, hay, straw	Vet and med, farrier	Wages	Rent, rates, property	Vehicle and power exps	Office and admin exps	Loan repay-ment	Private drawings	VAT on inputs	VAT to C&E	Value of inputs
01/05	Brought forward		13,135.03	1,560.00	320.00	2,330.00	3,699.00	174.00	386.00	1,000.00	680.00	452.03	2,534.00	6,139.00
12/05	District Council	121	286.00				286.00							
17/05	BT – phone	122	192.70						164.00			28.70		164.00
22/05	Compton Times ad.	123	82.25						70.00			12.25		70.00
27/05	Wages	124	2,330.00			2,330.00								
27/05	Private drawings	125	620.00								620.00			
31/05	Feed supplies	126	720.00	720.00										720.00
31/05	B. Smith – farrier	127	217.38		185.00							32.38		185.00
31/05	T. Tile – roof reps.	128	119.00				119.00							119.00
	Total for May		4,567.33	720.00	185.00	2,330.00	405.00	0.00	234.00	0.00	620.00	73.33	0.00	1,258.00
	Cum. total Apr–May		17,702.36	2,280.00	505.00	4,660.00	4,104.00	174.00	620.00	1,000.00	1,300.00	525.36	2,534.00	7,397.00

Figure 3.10 Oxhill Stables – cash analysis book – payments

Exercise_____

Obtain two sheets of accounts paper.

(1) Linda's transactions for June are shown below.

Use the column headings shown in the example for May. On the top row enter the totals brought forward from the end of May, then enter the details for June.

Date	Detail	(£) total
Receipts		
1/6	B. Black – livery fee £226.30, £12 sundry, plus £41.70 VAT	280.00
6/6	Lessons for week commencing 1/6 £1,730 inc. VAT	1,730.00
8/6	M. Smith – livery £124.58, sundry £15, plus £24.42 VAT	164.00
13/6	Lessons for week commencing 8/6, £1,776 inc. VAT	1,776.00
20/6	Lessons for week commencing 15/6, £1,812 inc. VAT	1,812.00
23/6	M. Blenkinsop – livery fee £271.49 + VAT	319.00
25/6	H. Jump – livery fee £73.20 + VAT	86.00
27/6	Lessons for week commencing 22/6, £1,895 inc. VAT	1,895.00
Payments		
12/6	Midshire District Council – rates	286.00
19/6	Compton Times – advert, £85 + VAT	99.88
26/6	Wages	2,300.00
26/6	Private drawings	580.00
30/6	Feed supplies – hard feeds, £520	520.00
30/6	Jab & Hope – vet, £224.60 + VAT	263.91
30/6	Jack Straw – bedding, £400 (no VAT)	400.00
30/6	Spanner & Bodgit – van repairs, £125 + VAT	146.88
30/6	Bank charges	68.50

(2) From the column totals for the quarter April to June, work out the figures that need to be included in the following VAT return boxes:

(a) VAT due on sales and other outputs
(b) VAT reclaimed on purchases and other inputs
(c) Net VAT to be paid to Customs and Excise (difference between a and b)
(d) Total value of sales and other outputs
(e) Total value of purchases and other inputs.

Chapter 4
Called to Account
The Main Accounts Documents

It is a legal requirement that the business produces a set of accounts each year. This allows the tax authorities to assess how much tax is due from the business or its owner. An accountant is usually employed to prepare the accounts, so that both the manager and tax inspector can have confidence that the figures are correct.

The annual set of accounts consists of two main documents:

- ❏ the trading and profit and loss account
- ❏ balance sheets for the start and end of the year.

Balance Sheet

The aim of a balance sheet is to show what a business is worth on a particular date. This involves adding up the value of all the assets that the business owns, and all of its liabilities or debts. The difference between assets and liabilities is called the net capital. This represents the value of the business to the owner – if all the assets were sold and all debts settled, this is how much money would be left.

Assets minus liabilities = net capital

The assets of a business will always be balanced by the liabilities plus net capital, as shown in Figure 4.1.

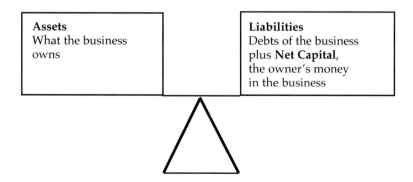

Assets	Liabilities
What the business	Debts of the business
owns	plus **Net Capital**,
	the owner's money
	in the business

Figure 4.1   The balance of assets and liabilities

On the balance sheets prepared by an accountant, both assets and liabilities are divided into different categories.

Assets

Fixed assets

Fixed assets are the long-term assets of the business in which money is invested for a number of years, such as property, vehicles, breeding and school horses. Their main purpose is to produce the goods and services of the business, rather than to be sold themselves.

Current assets

Current assets are stocks of goods (including horses) for sale, or materials such as feed used in the course of production. Also included here are the money assets, bank balances and debtors (sums of money owed to the business by customers).

Current assets are sometimes called circulating assets, because they are quickly changed from stocks to cash and back to stocks again (Figure 4.2).

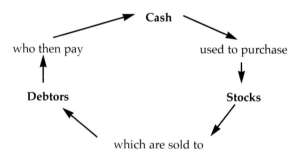

Figure 4.2   The cycle of current assets (money cycle)

On the balance sheet, assets are listed with the most difficult to convert to cash at the top, and ready money at the bottom – the inverse order of liquidity.

Liabilities

Current liabilities

Current liabilities are the short-term (up to one year) borrowings of the business, such as bank overdraft and creditors (sums owed to suppliers).

Long-term liabilities

Other debts are listed as long-term liabilities.

Net current assets

This is an extra figure shown on the balance sheet, and is sometimes called the working capital. This is because it is the amount of money that the business has available to continue its normal working activities. It is calculated by the formula:

Net current assets = current assets minus current liabilities

Running short of working capital is a common business problem, hence the importance of showing the net current assets figure on the balance sheet.

Balance sheet layout

The set of accounts for a financial year contains two balance sheets; one for the start and one for the end of the year. The date is important as the balance sheet always applies to a specific point in time. A typical balance sheet is shown in Figure 4.3.

To calculate the net capital figure:

Net capital = (fixed assets plus current assets)
minus (current plus long-term liabilities)

or

Net capital = fixed assets plus net current assets minus long-term liabilities

The 'Financed by' section at the bottom of the balance sheet is to explain why the value of the business has changed over the year. It may have been increased by the business making a profit, or decreased by private drawings having been taken out by the owner.

Negative figures are usually shown in accounts in parentheses. Hence (11,780) is the same as –11,780.

Trading and Profit and Loss Account

This shows the profit that the business has made from its activities, over a specific period of time. It usually relates to the financial year of the business.

What is profit?

Profit is an important concept in business management, as a business cannot survive if it does not make any. However it is often misunderstood. For example, during a financial year a dealing yard:

buys 20 horses for £30,000
sells 20 horses for £50,000
other costs total £10,000

Windmill Stables – balance sheet on 31 March 199_

	£	£
Fixed assets		
Buildings and fixtures	15,360	
Machinery and vehicles	11,400	
Brood mares	3,000	
		29,760
Current assets		
Young horses	10,800	
Stores of feed	250	
Debtors	2,240	
Bank balance	200	
	13,490	
Current liabilities		
Creditors	1,420	
Bank overdraft	3,202	
	4,622	
Net current assets		**8,868**
Long-term liability		
Bank loan		3,000
Net capital		**35,628**
Financed by:		
Opening net capital		34,380
Add: net profit for the year		13,028
		47,408
Subtract: private drawings		(11,780)
		35,628

Figure 4.3   Balance sheet for Windmill Stables

To work out the profit:

	£	£
Sales		50,000
Less costs		
Horses	30,000	
Other	10,000	
		40,000
Profit		**10,000**

Here the profit is the difference between the income and expenses of the business. Reality is usually more complicated however.
    Say the business had:

Five horses at the start of the year worth £7,500
Eight at the end of the year worth £12,000.

During the year it:

buys 23 horses for £35,000
sells 20 horses for £50,000
other costs total £10,000

The change in value of horses owned between the start and end of the year now needs to be included in the profit calculation.

	£	£
Sales		50,000
Change in value of horses:		
Closing value	12,000	
Opening value	7,500	
		4,500
		54,500
Less costs		
Horses	35,000	
Other	10,000	
		45,000
Profit		**9,500**

So profit can be, and usually is, more than the difference between income and expenses. It can be defined as:

'The difference in value between the outputs of a business and its inputs over a given time period.'

Outputs are what the business produces and sells *out*; inputs are what goes *in* to producing the sales, such as feed, labour, etc. The stock at the start of the year is an input into the accounting period, and that which is left at the end is an output to the next period. This is illustrated in Figure 4.4.

The trading and profit and loss account is calculated in two stages.

Trading account

The trading account shows what the business has sold during the period, and the direct costs involved in producing those sales.

Sales minus cost of sales = gross profit

The gross profit is not just about money received. Part of the profit can be in extra stocks at the end of the year.

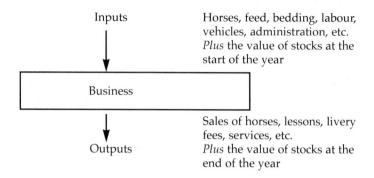

Inputs

Horses, feed, bedding, labour,
vehicles, administration, etc.
Plus the value of stocks at the
start of the year

Business

Outputs

Sales of horses, lessons, livery
fees, services, etc.
Plus the value of stocks at the
end of the year

Figure 4.4   Business inputs and outputs

Cost of sales = opening stock plus direct costs minus closing stock

An example could be in a dealing yard. The business starts the year with four
horses. During the year it buys twelve horses but only sells ten. It therefore
has six horses at the end of the year.

Four horses at the start of the year (opening stock)
Twelve horses purchased

Dealing yard

Ten horses sold
Six horses left at the end of the year (closing stock)

The trading account for this situation, with financial data included, will be:

			£
Sales	10 horses @ £3,000		30,000
Cost of sales			
Direct costs	12 horses purchased @ £2,000	24,000	
Plus opening stock	4 horses @ £2,000	8,000	
		32,000	
Less closing stock	6 horses @ £2,000	(12,000)	
			20,000
Gross profit			10,000

Profit and loss account

The profit and loss account takes the gross profit from the trading account,
and adds any income from sources other than sales, such as interest and

rents received. Then, to arrive at the bottom line net profit, the overhead expenses of the business such as rent, rates, labour, etc. are deducted.

Net profit = gross profit plus other income minus overhead expenses

The trading account and profit and loss account are usually combined under the one heading of trading and profit and loss account. A typical example, to complete the accounts for Windmill Stables, is shown in Figure 4.5.

Windmill Stables – trading and profit and loss account for the year ending 31 March 199_

	£	£
Sales		
Livery fees	52,710	
Sales of youngsters	12,400	
Sundry livery income	3,540	
		68,650
Less cost of sales		
Opening stock	12,400	
Feed	7,554	
Bedding	3,684	
Hay	6,286	
Veterinary and medicines	890	
Farriery	120	
Stud fees and mare's livery	1,020	
	31,954	
Less closing stock	(14,050)	
		17,904
Gross profit		**50,746**
Overheads		
Paid labour	15,288	
Rent	7,000	
Rates and water	2,800	
Machinery and vehicles expenses	6,160	
Contractors – grassland maintenance	400	
Property repairs and maintenance	1,620	
Insurance	980	
Accountancy	800	
Office and administration expenses	1,700	
Bank interest and charges	970	
		37,718
Net profit for the year		**13,028**

Figure 4.5   Trading and profit and loss account for Windmill Stables

The net profit figure here is the same as that shown in the 'Financed by' section of the balance sheet, thus providing a link between the two documents.

Exercises _____

(1) A stables business has the following assets and liabilities on 31 October 199_:

	£
Premises	250,000
Brood mares	8,000
Vehicles	14,000
Young horses	9,000
Debtors	500
Cash	50
Mortgage	50,000
Trade creditors	1,200
Bank overdraft	5,000

Draw up the balance sheet, using the format illustrated earlier in this chapter.

(2) During the year ending 31 October 199_, the business had:

	£
Sales of	£80,000
Direct costs of	£20,000
Overhead expenses of	£45,000
Value of stocks on 30 October	£9,000
Value of opening stocks on 1 November	£7,000

Calculate the gross profit and net profit for the year.

(3) The business had opening net capital of £218,350
Private drawings during the year were £10,000

Use this information to complete the 'Financed by' section at the bottom of the balance sheet.

_____

Chapter 5
Another Year Over
The Financial Year End

At the end of each financial year, all of the records of the business need to be brought together and the accounts prepared. This is quite complicated, and often involves ploughing through a box full of papers and books. Many business owners do not relish the task and leave it to a qualified accountant.

The aim of this chapter is to create awareness of the work done by accountants, not to make them redundant. They are important allies to a business:

❑   making sure that all of the figures end up in the right place
❑   giving valuable advice to the manager on financial and taxation matters.

Also the tax authorities are less likely to question accounts prepared by a professional.

The box load of information that will need to be sent to the accountant consists of:

❑   The completed cash analysis book for the year, or computer 'audit trail' printout detailing all transactions.
❑   All invoices, cheque book stubs, bank statements, receipts, and other documents relating to transactions.
❑   A list of debtors and creditors at both the start and end of the year.
❑   Valuation of all the assets of the business at the end of the year, and balance sheet for the start of the year.

The first stage in preparing the accounts is to go through all of the records to check that everything has been recorded correctly. After this the amounts can be totalled and the trading and profit and loss account and balance sheet drawn up.

Trading and Profit and Loss (TP&L) Account

Most of the information for the trading and profit and loss account is taken from the cash analysis book. A few important changes have to be made to the cash analysis book figures, and one or two other pieces of information have to be included.

Private and capital items

The key word in the title of the account is 'trading'. This means that it needs to show what the business has made from its on-going activities. Any private or capital sums in the cash analysis book therefore need to be left out of the TP&L account. VAT amounts are also excluded.
  Private items include:

❏   private drawings for the owner's living expenses;
❏   income tax payments;
❏   a proportion of the telephone and electricity bills, if the business and private accommodation are not separately invoiced;
❏   costs of keeping horses for personal use – including feed, veterinary, farrier expenses, and labour costs – should also be left out of the accounts. This is an area that can easily cause problems, for example if a horse is used for both business and private uses.

Capital items are investments in assets such as premises, buildings or vehicles, or sales of such assets. Any monies concerned with loans, except interest payments, are also left out of the TP&L account.

Depreciation

Depreciation is a sum to allow for the loss in value of an asset over time, through age, use or obsolescence. It is included in the accounts as an overhead expense, instead of the full cost of capital assets. In this way, the cost of such assets is spread over a number of years.
  For example, if a yard invested £20,000 in a new horse box, the figure entered in the TP&L account would be the depreciation, to reflect the fall in value of the box over the year, not the £20,000 purchase price.
  The basis for calculating depreciation depends on the nature of the assets.

Reducing balance

The reducing balance method is usually used for vehicles and machinery. Each year, the value of the asset is reduced by a percentage of its value at the start of the year. To continue with the horse box example from above, and using a depreciation rate of 25%, Table 5.1 shows that the depreciation, or decline in value, is less each year as the asset ages.

Table 5.1   Calculating depreciation on a horse box

Year	Cost £	Depreciation for year £	Closing value £
1	20,000	5,000	15,000
2		3,750	11,250
3		2,813	8,437
4		2,109	6,328

Straight line

Buildings and fixtures are depreciated on the straight line basis. Here the loss in value each year remains the same – a percentage of the original cost. Table 5.2 shows as an example, an outdoor arena costing £25,000 and depreciated at 4% per year.

Table 5.2   Calculating depreciation on an arena

Year	Cost	Depreciation for year	Closing value
	£	£	£
1	25,000	1,000	24,000
2		1,000	23,000
3		1,000	22,000
4		1,000	21,000

If these figures are drawn on a graph, the value of the asset declines in a straight line, and will reach zero after 25 years. This is illustrated in Figure 5.1.

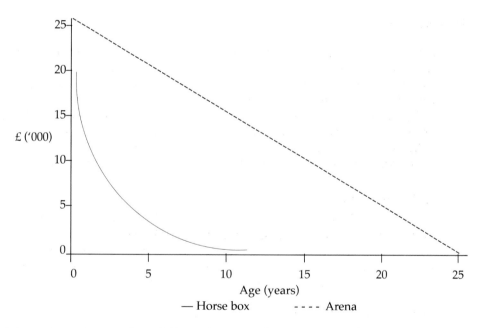

— Horse box   - - - - Arena

Figure 5.1   Straight line and reducing balance depreciation

A section showing how depreciation has been calculated is usually included in the accounts, under the heading 'Schedule of fixed assets'.

Opening and closing stock

Opening and closing stock will include the value of any stocks of materials such as feed or bedding, and horses.

A major principle of accounting is the prudence concept, which states that a profit should not be anticipated. Stocks are therefore valued at the lower of either their:

❑ original cost, *or*
❑ net realisable value (what they could be sold for, less the cost of selling them).

The same basis of valuation should be used for items from year to year. The services of a professional valuer may be employed to prepare the valuation.

Debtors and creditors adjustments

The TP&L account needs to show the value of goods bought or sold during the year. The cash analysis book, however, states the money received or paid for different items. In some circumstances these are not the same. For example, a stables may have sold £10,000 worth of livery services, and this is the amount that should be included in the TP&L account. If £1,000 is still owed by the customers, the cash analysis book will only show that £9,000 has been received.

Where there are debtors or creditors at either end of the year, the cash analysis book totals need adjusting. This is done by adding the closing debtor/creditor, and subtracting the opening figure. Say a feed bill was unpaid at each end of the year:

	Feed (£)
Cash analysis book total	8,000
+ Closing creditor	900
– Opening creditor	(700)
Total for TP&L account	8,200

The closing creditor is money that has not yet been paid, but needs to be accounted for in the current year, whereas the opening creditor is money paid in this financial year but which was accounted for last year. Hence the value of feed bought in the year is £8,200, not the £8,000 recorded as paid in the cash analysis book. This is illustrated in Figure 5.2.

Drawing up the account

Having gathered all of the data, checked it, and made the necessary adjustments, the TP&L account can then be drawn up in the format described in the previous chapter.

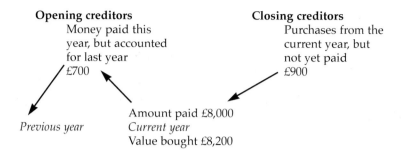

Figure 5.2 Creditor adjustments

Balance Sheet

A balance sheet for the start of the year will be available from last year's accounts. The data for the closing balance sheet needs to be drawn together.

Assets

- ❏ Premises – based on historic cost, which is the price originally paid when they were bought.
- ❏ Buildings, machinery, vehicles and equipment – the value after depreciation has been deducted.
- ❏ Stocks – the valuation considered above.
- ❏ Debtors – amounts owed by customers.
- ❏ Bank balance and cash on hand.

Liabilities

- ❏ Creditors – money owed to suppliers and others.
- ❏ Overdraft – the overdrawn bank balance.
- ❏ Loans and mortgages – the outstanding balance on the accounts.

Case Study

The following shows the process of preparing Linda's accounts for the year ending 31 March 1996. It should be borne in mind that understanding the content of the finalised accounts is more important than knowing the detail of how they are put together.

Information required

(1) Cash analysis book totals for the year

These are shown in Figures 5.3 and 5.4, together with the necessary adjustments for debtors and creditors to give the totals for the accounts.

(2) Balance sheet on 31 March 1995

	£	£
Fixed assets		
Buildings	19,200	
Vehicles	6,000	
Horses and ponies	21,500	
Tack and equipment	4,500	
		51,200
Current assets		
Feed stocks	190	
Debtors	170	
	360	
Current liabilities		
Creditors	120	
Bank overdraft	19,495	
	19,615	
Net current assets		**(19,255)**
Long-term liabilities		
Loan		16,000
Net capital		**15,945**

(3) Debtors and creditors

Opening debtor (livery)	£170
Closing debtor (livery)	£350
Opening creditor (feed)	£120
Closing creditor (feed)	£155

(4) Valuations on 31 March 1996

Horses and ponies	£18,900
Feed stocks	£220

(5) Bank balance on 31 March 1996

£1,849 overdrawn

Procedure for preparing the accounts

1)   Totals for TP&L account from the cash analysis book

Adjustments for debtors and creditors, and items to be excluded from the account, are shown in Figures 5.3 and 5.4.

(2) Opening and closing stock

From the balance sheet for 31 March 1995, the opening stock is:

	£
Horses and ponies	21,500
Feed stocks	190
	21,690

The valuation figures for 31 March 1996 give a closing stock sum of £19,120.

(3) Depreciation

A value needs to be calculated for buildings and vehicles.

Buildings:	£
Initial cost	20,000
Value on 31/3/95	19,200
Depreciation (4%, straight line)	800
Value on 31/3/96	18,400

Vehicles:	£
Value on 31/3/95	6,000
Depreciation (25%, reducing balance)	1,500
Value on 31/3/96	4,500

(4) Draw up the trading and profit and loss account

The sums are now all available to draw up in the format described in the previous chapter.

(5) Complete the closing balance sheet

All of the data needed for this has also been prepared and can be arranged in the correct manner.

The completed accounts are shown in Figures 5.5 and 5.6. They should be examined carefully to see how the figures have been derived from the information above.

Detail	Riding lessons	Livery fees	Sundry income	VAT on sales
Total for year	85,276.00	19,582.00	2,450.00	18,818.00
Opening debtor		-170.00		
Closing debtor		350.00		
Accounts total	85,276.00	19,762.00	2,450.00	—

Figure 5.3   Oxhill Stables – cash analysis book – receipts

Detail	Conc. feed	Hay	Straw	Farrier	Vet. and med.	Grass exps.	Wages and NI	Rent	Rates	Water	Electric	Vehicle exps.
Total for year	9,368.00	6,486.00	3,347.00	2,380.00	1,390.00	275.00	27,980.00	8,000.00	3,060.00	560.00	438.00	269.00
Opening creditor	-120.00											
Closing creditor	155.00											
Accounts total	9,403.00	6,486.00	3,347.00	2,380.00	1,390.00	275.00	27,980.00	8,000.00	3,060.00	560.00	438.00	2,690.00

Detail	Property repairs	Tack repairs	Insurance	Advert.	Phone& office	Bank int. ch.	Loan interest	Loan repay	Private tax	VAT on inputs	VAT to C&E
Total for year	1,230.00	1,322.00	2,310.00	724.00	1,774.00	1,758.00	2,240.00	4,000.00	8,340.00	3,526.25	15,284.15
Accounts total	1,230.00	1,322.00	2,310.00	724.00	1,774.00	1,758.00	2,240.00	—	—	—	—

Figure 5.4   Oxhill Stables – cash analysis book – payments

Miss L. Clark, Oxhill Stables
Accounts for the year ending 31 March 1996
Balance sheet

	31 March 96		1 April 95	
	£	£	£	£
Fixed assets				
Buildings	18,400		19,200	
Vehicles	4,500		6,000	
Horses and ponies	18,900		21,500	
Tack and equipment	4,500		4,500	
		46,300		51,200
Current assets				
Feed stocks	220		190	
Debtors	350		170	
Bank balance				
	570		360	
Current liabilities				
Creditors	155		120	
Bank overdraft	1,849		19,495	
	2,004		19,615	
Net current assets		**(1,434)**		**(19,255)**
Long-term liabilities				
Bank loan		12,000		16,000
Net capital		**32,866**		**15,945**
Financed by:				
Net capital on 1/4/95		15,945		
+ net profit		25,261		
– private and tax		(8,340)		
Net capital on 31/3/96		**32,866**		

Schedule of fixed assets

	Initial cost	Value on 1/4/95	Deprec- iation	Deprec- iation	Value on 31/3/96
	£	£	%	£	£
Buildings	20,000	19,200	4	800	18,400
Vehicles		6,000	25	1,500	4,500

Figure 5.5   Balance sheet for Oxhill Stables

Miss L. Clark, Oxhill Stables
Trading and profit and loss account for the year ending 31 March 1996

	£	£
Sales		
Riding lessons	85,276	
Livery fees	19,762	
Sundry livery income	2,450	
		107,488
Less cost of sales		
Opening stock	21,690	
Concentrate feed	9,403	
Hay	6,486	
Straw	3,347	
Farrier	2,380	
Veterinary and medicines	1,390	
Grassland expenses	275	
	44,971	
Less closing stock	(19,120)	
		25,851
Gross profit		**81,637**
Overheads		
Wages and NI		27,980
Rent		8,000
Rates		3,060
Water		560
Electricity		438
Vehicle expenses		2,680
Vehicle depreciation		1,500
Property repairs and maintenance		1,230
Buildings depreciation		800
Tack repairs and replacement		1,322
Insurance		2,310
Advertising		724
Telephone, office expenses and fees		1,774
Loan interest		2,240
Bank interest and charges		1,758
		56,376
Net profit		**25,261**

Figure 5.6   Trading and profit and loss account for Oxhill Stables

Part 2

Ours is the Future

Planning and Budgeting

Chapter 6
Ideas and Numbers
Introducing Planning and Budgeting

A business venture will always begin with ideas. Planning involves the development of these ideas so that they can be put into practice. To accompany these plans, budgets need to be prepared to work out costs and likely income. This process is a part of normal life. For example, it could be the idea for a summer holiday in the sun. Possible resorts are researched, and plans are then developed to go to a certain place. To accompany these plans, calculations are made about the likely costs of travel, accommodation, spending money, etc., what value of travellers' cheques are needed. These become the budget for the holiday – numbers to go with the ideas.

Hence planning is the development of ideas; budgets are the numbers (in financial terms) to evaluate the plans. It can be expressed conveniently as a cycle – the planning cycle (Figure 6.1).

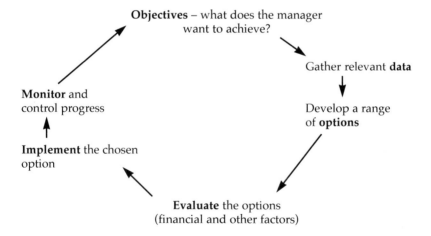

Figure 6.1   The planning cycle

Planning Cycle

Objectives

The starting point is to ask, 'What do I want to achieve in and through the business?' These objectives can be financial or personal. Possible examples are shown in Figure 6.2.

Personal	*Financial*
Lifestyle – able to compete or hunt	Achieve a certain standard of living
Freedom of being own boss	Make maximum profit
Ambition to succeed	Return on capital
Reputation for quality	
Growth	

Figure 6.2   Business objectives

The main objective of any business must be financial. At a minimum, this would be to make enough profit to be viable, i.e. to provide the owner with an acceptable standard of living, as well as maintaining the assets of the business and repaying any borrowed money. If this minimum financial requirement cannot be met then any objectives of ambition, lifestyle, etc. will certainly not be fulfilled, as the business will be unable to continue.

Options and data

The options will be business ideas that might satisfy the objectives already identified. To see if this will be the case a quantity of data is required, which will cover a number of areas, such as finance, legislation and marketing.
  Market information is discussed in the next chapter.

Legal aspects

The law is a complex area beyond the scope of this book, and a number of texts have been written specifically on the subject of horses and the law. Further to these, a solicitor's advice is often helpful. It is important to find out about any legal requirements before starting a business, to avoid possible trouble later. A few examples of legal aspects that may need to be considered are:

❑   insurance cover, for public and employer's liability;
❑   planning permission may be needed for the establishment or expansion of premises, or change of use;
❑   the requirements of the Health and Safety at Work Act;
❑   the Riding Establishments Act could be relevant.

Financial data

The most important source of financial data for planning an existing business is its own information on costs, levels of sales, etc. This will be the most reliable guide for preparing future budgets.
  For the new business, or one developing into new areas, external sources of information are needed. Various possibilities are given here.

Suppliers
Suppliers can provide costs for feed, buildings, etc. Insurance companies can give quotations for the necessary cover for a given situation; similarly electricity and water companies can give likely costs for a business venture, if provided with appropriate details. An indication of business rates can be obtained from the local authority.

Reference books
The major text on horse business financial data is the *Equine Business Guide*, published jointly by Warwickshire College, Moreton Morrell, Warwick and the Welsh Institute of Rural Studies, Aberystwyth. This contains details of typical costs and returns for a wide range of equine enterprises, derived from a survey of a large number of horse businesses.

Consultants and professional advisers
When starting a new business it is advisable to make full use of the expertise of others, such as accountants, Department of Trade and Industry small business advisers, and the bank manager. A number of consultants specialise in horse businesses.

Evaluate

Having gathered all the data together it is time to work out whether the ideas are likely to be successful financially. This involves preparing various budgets, details of which are found in chapters 8–11.

Implement

The chosen plan is now put into action.

Monitor and control

It is important that all the plans and budgets are not just left to gather dust at this stage. Instead the progress of the business needs to be monitored against the budgets, so that the manager can see if everything is going according to plan. If problems arise (or when, which is more likely), they can be quickly spotted, and appropriate action taken. This is the basis of budgetary control, which is covered in more detail in chapter 12.

Risk and Uncertainty

Implicit in all that has been written is that planning and budgeting involve looking into the future. This can never be done with perfect knowledge, which is part of the challenge. Unexpected events can always arise, and may adversely affect the business. A number of these factors that can influence the horse business are shown in Figure 6.3.

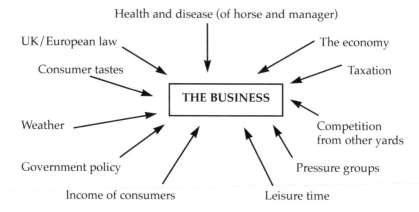

Figure 6.3   External influences on a horse business

With so many factors that can upset the best of plans, the question could be asked – are the planning and budgeting worth all the effort? Compare starting a new business venture to a mountaineer heading off into mist enshrouded hills. He or she would be considered most unwise to go without a map and compass to guide them. Their chances of reaching the destination with nothing to navigate by are much reduced; rather they are more likely to get lost, or worse.

For a business, the plans and budgets are the tools with which to navigate into the clouds of uncertainty that lie ahead. The chances of success are much greater with them than without. Too many new businesses get lost in the early stages of the journey, and poor planning is often a major factor.

Chapter 7
Getting it Down on Paper
The Business Plan

To get a business idea off the ground requires a great deal more than inspiration. A lot of research is needed, and this all needs to be condensed into a clear and ordered presentation. The business plan is the way to achieve this in a manner which will show that the proposals are sensible and viable.

Preparing a business plan is useful to:

❑ A new business – the plan will need to outline resources and facilities needed, establish that a market demand exists, detail the finance required and show that the business will be profitable.
❑ An existing business seeking to develop or expand, or one that wants to look at future possibilities. The plan also provides working guidelines for the management and the direction of the business over the coming period.
❑ Support a request to borrow money – many business plans are prepared at the bank manager's insistence.

Once the plan has been prepared, it should not be considered as 'cast in tablets of stone' and unchangeable. Rather, it should be reviewed at least every three months and updated in the light of progress and the prevailing state of affairs.

Guides and outlines to assist with preparing the business plan are available from banks and other organisations. These help to make sure that all of the relevant points are covered. It is important that the plan is presented in a clear and attractive way, to give a positive first impression to any readers.

The Business Plan

A typical business plan will consist of a number of sections:

Contents

These should be listed, with page numbers, so that anyone unfamiliar with the plan can quickly find their way around.

Introduction

This will briefly state the type of business, its location, premises, and any funding requirements.

Business proposals

Include the objectives of the business and a description of the activities to be pursued. The legal format to be adopted should also be mentioned, i.e. whether the business will be run as a sole trader, partnership or limited company.

Marketing

This is a very important section of the plan, and will itself need to cover a number of factors.

Target market

A description of the target market should be included – that is, the type of customers the business will hope to attract and where they are to be found.

Demand

An assessment should be made of the demand for the product or service, and whether this is rising, static or in decline. It is often hard to give specific information on this, but an awareness of the current state of the industry is important.

Competition

This covers who the competition are and where they operate. It is necessary to research similar yards in the area to try and get an idea of the services they offer, prices charged, and any strengths or weaknesses that the proposal may have compared to them. Some information about competitor businesses can be found in references such as Yellow Pages, Thompsons Directory, BHS *Where To Ride*, British Equestrian Directory, etc. However, there will always be some yards that are not listed in any of these places, so there is no substitute for local knowledge and keeping an ear to the ground.

Promotional strategy

Promotional strategy is more than placing advertisements. The business can be promoted in many other ways, such as by entering competitions or shows, open days, or sending press releases to local papers. If these are well worded and accompanied by a good photograph they will often be printed, especially for a new business, providing valuable free advertising.

Formal advertising remains a very important tool of marketing, so appropriate publications, local or national depending upon the type of business, should be considered, along with their costs. The vital decision is which will be the most cost effective for reaching the potential customers.

Pricing policy

The price level to charge may be set by considering the competition and matching, or undercutting, them. It is often better to try and compete on quality and service, rather than price cutting. An alternative is to calculate the costs of providing a service such as lessons or livery, and then add a profit margin on top – 'cost plus pricing'. It is important that a price worked out in this way is still competitive in the marketplace.

Resource requirements

Included here will be details of the premises and any improvements or modifications needed; also any vehicles, machinery or equipment and horses that will be bought. Costs for all of these items need to be estimated.

Personnel

The owner/manager is a vital person in the running of a business. Their qualifications and experience which make them suitable for the position should be emphasised. An up-to-date curriculum vitae can be included as an appendix to the plan. Similar details for any other key members of staff already employed (for example a head girl/lad), should also be included.

Other staff required by the business should be listed, including their job title, a brief job description, qualifications or experience required, and pay.

When planning the number of staff to employ it is important to allow for days off and holidays. Part time or casual help should be considered, as well as full time workers. There are limits to both the availability and capability of working pupils and trainees, so they should not be relied on too heavily in the staffing plan.

It is a significant advantage to have some staff living on the yard, for security and emergency reasons.

Finance

This is the most important area of the plan, and needs to include:

❑   Details of recent financial performance, if the business is already trading. The accounts for the past three years should be sufficient.
❑   A new or expanding business will need to detail set-up costs, such as property, buildings and horses. These are the one-off expenses that are

needed to get the business started.
- ❏ Budgets to show that the proposals will make a sufficiently high level of profit to be viable and repay any borrowing.
- ❏ Financial forecasts, certainly for the next year, and possibly for two or three years. These budgets will take the form of profit forecasts, cash flows, and perhaps projected balance sheets.

The detail of preparing these budgets can be found in chapters 8–11.

Conclusions

These will draw together the main points of the preceding sections.

Appendices

The main text of the plan should 'flow', without being cluttered up by complex calculations, lists or inventories. These should be summarised in the text, and the reader then referred to an appendix where the material can be presented in detail.

Case Study

Background

At the beginning of 1994, Linda Clark was 23 and had been involved with horses for many years. She had worked in several yards, completed a National Diploma in Horse Studies course at an agricultural college, and recently gained her BHS Intermediate Instructor certificate.

Her father owns a farm, and was prepared to make available to Linda a building measuring 20 m by 30 m for use as an indoor school. The farm already had six stables, and Linda could develop more. She could also have the use of 4 har (10 acres) of grassland.

With her own money and a sum that her father made available, Linda had £20,000 to develop her business. She prepared the following business plan to support her request for a loan from her local bank, and also to assess for herself whether her proposals were viable and feasible.

Note: the financial components of the plan are mentioned in the following text but can be found in later chapters. In reality, the budgets would be included at the appropriate point in the plan.

Contents

Business Plan

Miss Linda Clark

Oxhill Stables
Oxhill Farm
Nether Compton
Midshire
NC10 4TF
(01623) 123456

January 1994

Introduction

This business plan sets out proposals for the development of a riding school and livery business at Oxhill Farm, Nether Compton, which is owned by Mr P. Clark.

The business will be operated and managed by Miss Linda Clark as sole trader, but with the financial support of the family. A rent of £8,000 per year will be payable for the use of the premises, which consist of a building measuring 20 m by 30 m, plus six stables and 10 acres of grazing.

Oxhill Farm is located four miles from the town of Nether Compton (population 160,000) and two miles from Windmarsh (population 5,000). It is easily accessible from the B1640 and the main motorway network.

Development of the business will require investment of £20,000 in building works and £31,000 in horses, ponies and tack. £20,000 of personal and family finance is available, plus vehicles to the value of £8,000. The support of the bank is requested in the form of a loan for £20,000 and an overdraft facility of £26,000 in the first year of trading. Oxhill Farm can be offered as security for any borrowing.

Business Proposals

Objectives

(1) To develop a successful business with a reputation for quality service.
(2) To generate sufficient cash surplus to repay borrowed money within five years and support an acceptable standard of living. A figure of £10,000 per year is required.
(3) To improve personal skills and success in competitions.

Facilities

Details of the existing and proposed facilities are:

Existing: 20 m × 30 m indoor school
                       6 brick built stables

Proposed: 10 new timber stables, plus feed and
                       tack rooms
                       Improvements to indoor school

Activities

The business will be based upon two main activities, a riding school and livery service.

(1) Riding school

It is planned to own six ponies for giving lessons to children aged 6–14 years, and eight horses suitable for training older teenagers and adults up to BHS stage 2 standard. Supervised hacks along local bridleways will also be conducted.

Proposed charges (inclusive of VAT) are:

Children's group lesson   £6.50/half hour
Adults' group lesson   £12.00/hour
Private lessons   £14.00/hour
Hack   £10.00/hour

In year two it is assumed that ponies will be used for 10 hours per week on average, mainly at weekends, summer evenings and during school holidays. Use of the horses is expected to be 14 hours per week and subject to less seasonality.

Expected income in 1995/96 (exclusive of VAT):

	£
Children's lessons	30,536
Adults' lessons/hacks	52,616
	83,152
% of total turnover	77

(2) Livery service

This will provide a full service, including feeding, mucking out, grooming and exercise. The charge will be £75 (inclusive of VAT) per week, payable in advance.

Additional services such as instruction, transport and clipping will be available to clients.

Eight boxes are available for this service. Uptake of the facility is assumed to be 45 weeks in 1995/6, giving a total income (excluding VAT) of:

	£
Livery fees	22,979
Additional services	2,000
	24,979
% of total turnover	23

Statutory Matters

It is proposed to start business on 1 April 1994.

Planning permission has been obtained from the District Council for change of use of the premises from agricultural to equine use. A licence to operate as a riding school under the Riding Establishments Acts (1964 and 1970) has been applied for.

3

Personal Details

Name:	Linda Jane Clark
Address:	Oxhill Farm
	Nether Compton
	Midshire
	NC10 4TF
Telephone:	(01623) 123456
Date of birth:	23 September 1970
Qualifications:	BTEC National Diploma in Horse Studies (Distinction)
	Warwickshire College, Moreton Morrell, Warks. 1992
	British Horse Society Intermediate Instructor (BHS II). 1993
Work experience:	Sept 1992–Jan 1994
	Stanton Equestrian Centre, Stanton, Essex
	A leading training centre in the East of England. Head girl for the last 14 months, in charge of day-to-day running of the yard and supervision of staff.
	July 1990–Aug 1991
	Mrs J. Rumple,
	Uttoxeter, Staffs.
	Event groom in a successful competition yard (Industrial Experience year of National Diploma course).
Personal qualities:	Organised, hard working and dedicated; gets on well with people; able to command respect and support of staff.

4

Other Staffing Requirements

It is envisaged that the following staff will be employed:

Assistant head girl
Qualified to BHS AI, to teach lessons and deputise for manager in day-to-day supervision of yard when necessary.

Four grooms
Qualified to BHS Stage 1 or 2 level. To provide daily care of the horses/ponies, prepare them for lessons, exercise livery horses.

Working pupil
Some experience with horses necessary, but will be trained towards BHS Stage 1 or 2. Assist grooms.

Weekend helper
Employed for six hours at weekends to assist with children's lessons and stable duties.

Wage levels

	£/week
Assistant head girl	130
Grooms	80
Working pupil	40
Weekend helper	30

Annual labour cost £27,040, plus £1,622 for employer's National Insurance contributions. Not all of these staff will be engaged immediately, but as the need arises.

5

The Market

(1) Riding school

This will be aimed towards the casual rider, wishing to learn to ride or improve, and children.

Competition

Two riding schools exist within a radius of 15 miles.

(a) Millthorpe Equestrian Centre is aimed at the more serious rider, and offers no service for young people. Charges range from £12/hour for a group lesson to £20/hour for a private lesson.

(b) Cobbly Stables is in a state of disrepair. It has no indoor school and a poor selection of mounts. Children's lessons are given, but the business is located further away from the major population centres of Nether Compton and Windmarsh. No hacks are conducted. Prices range from £6/half hour children's lesson to £10/hour for adults.

Reasons for supposing a market exists

(a) Lessons are being given to a clientele of 12 on a freelance basis, with enquiries received from other potential customers (six in the last two months).

(b) Involvement with the local Pony Club gives contact with a number of children who would like regular lessons, or who are dissatisfied with their existing arrangement.

(2) Livery service

This will be aimed at the horse owner who is unable to look after their own horse and requires a high quality, caring service.

6

Competition

Within a radius of 15 miles there are eight other establishments offering a livery service. These range from 'do-it-yourself' arrangements costing £10–18/week, to a full or specialised service costing £60–90/week.

Reasons for supposing a market exists

Four horses are already kept on livery at the farm, and eight enquiries have been received in the last six months.

(3) Marketing strategy

(a) The riding school will be publicised among the local Pony Clubs.
(b) Advertisements will be placed in local papers promoting the school and livery service. Adverts costing £20 each.
(c) Press releases with photographs will be sent to all local newspapers.
(d) People who have recently enquired about services will be contacted.

7

Financial Projections

(1) Establishment costs

Initial costs will consist of:

(a) Horses, ponies and tack

	£
6 ponies @ £1,200	7,200
8 horses @ £2,400	19,200
Tack for 14 mounts	4,500
	30,900

(b) Building works

Construction of 10 additional stables, feed and tack rooms, and improvements to indoor school. £20,000

(2) Financial potential of the business

Budgets detailed in appendices 1 and 2 indicate a potential net profit in excess of £20,000 per year. This is sufficient to achieve the objectives outlined earlier of private drawings totalling £10,000 per year and repayment of borrowed money within five years.

[*See chapter 8 for details of these budgets*]

8

(4) Projected balance sheets

These are shown in appendix 8, and summarised below:

Balance sheets on:	31/3/96	1/4/95	1/4/94
	£	£	£
Fixed assets	47,733	53,067	8,000
Current assets	0	0	20,000
Current liabilities	5,309	20,560	0
Net current assets	(5,309)	(20,560)	20,000
Long-term liability	12,000	16,000	0
Net capital	**30,424**	**16,507**	**28,000**

[*See chapter 12.*]

10

(3) Profit and cash flow forecasts for 1994/95 and 1995/96

The forecasts are detailed in appendices 3-6, and are summarised below:

	1994/5	1995/6
	£	£
Net profit (before interest on overdraft)	(1,279)	24,483
Bank overdraft interest	(2,214)	(1,565)
Net profit (loss)	(3,493)	22,918
Opening bank balance	20,000	(20,560)
Closing bank balance	(20,560)	(5,309)
Net cash flow	(40,560)	15,251
Peak overdraft requirement	26,000	25,000

Income during 1994/95 is assumed to be two thirds that of 1995/96. This is to allow for the developments of the property, which will take approximately two months, and for trade to be gradually built up. The small loss during this first year, accompanied by major establishment costs, result in the negative net cash flow. The overdraft is expected to peak at £26,000 in May, after which a gradual decline occurs for the remainder of the year.

Performance is expected to be much more satisfactory in 1995/6, with a healthy profit, and the overdraft reduced to £5,000 by the end of the year.

[*See chapter 9 for further details of the profit forecasts and chapter 10 for the cash flows.*]

Reconciliation of profit and cash flow forecasts is shown in appendix 7. [*See chapter 11.*]

9

Conclusions

Oxhill Farm is excellently situated for an equine business of the type proposed. Demand for services has already been identified through existing and potential customers. With the support of the bank in the form of a loan for £20,000 repayable over five years, and an overdraft facility of £26,000 for the first two years of trading, a profitable business can be established.

11

Chapter 8
Can the Ideas Work?
Budgeting Business Proposals

Budgets can take various forms. The first task is to assess the potential of a set of business ideas. How much profit are they capable of generating? Will it be enough for the business to succeed? Such a budget can be termed a system budget, as it seeks to show the profitability of an established business system which is operating at a normal level of trade. It allows the manager to assess whether the profit of the proposed business will provide an acceptable standard of living, and repay borrowing. An existing business may use it to compare the current system with alternative policies, to see if a change of direction is justified.

System Budget

The following stages are involved in compiling a system budget.

Prepare enterprise gross margin budgets

The business is divided into its different activities, such as livery horses of various types, dealing, teaching, shows and competitions, etc. These can be termed 'enterprises' or 'profit centres', each with readily identifiable items of sales and variable (or direct) costs. The gross margin budgets show, for each enterprise:

Sales minus variable costs = gross margin

The gross margin is how much gross profit each enterprise is contributing towards covering the overhead costs of the business, and to leave a net profit. The idea is illustrated in Figure 8.1.

An example of a gross margin budget, to show the typical content and layout, is given overleaf.

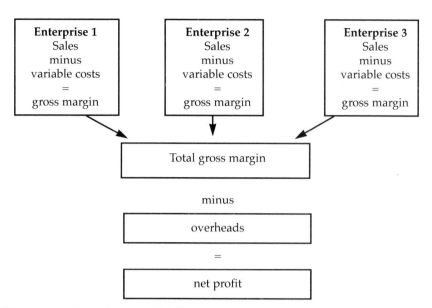

Figure 8.1 Contribution of different enterprises

Dealing horse	£
Sales	
Sale of horse	3,200
Variable costs	
Purchase of horse	2,000
Feed	60
Hay	50
Bedding	30
Veterinary and farrier	80
Marketing	120
	2,340
Gross margin per horse	**860**

Other examples are shown in the case study and in the appendix at the end of this chapter.

VAT in budgets

All figures in a budget should be exclusive of VAT, unless the business is not VAT registered, in which case VAT payable on different inputs should be included in the costs.

Total gross margin for the business

This is the sum of the enterprise gross margins. The plan should concentrate on the enterprises that produce a high gross margin, as this will lead to a high total gross margin, and hopefully net profit. Constraints of personal preference, finance, resources or market demand should be allowed for.

Example: A business has twelve stables available. The manager wishes to use

❑ two boxes for dealing, with eight horses brought and sold during a year and making £860 gross margin;
❑ ten boxes for full liveries – gross margin details below.

	£
Sales	
Livery fees	3,250
Variable costs	
Feed	400
Hay	200
Bedding	150
	750
Gross margin per livery	**2,500**

Some freelance teaching will also be undertaken. The total gross margin calculation is:

		£
Gross margins		
Full liveries	10 @ £2,500	25,000
Dealing horses	8 @ £860	6,880
Teaching 5 hours/week	@ £12	3,000
Total gross margin		**34,880**

Estimate overhead expenses

These are the costs that the business will have to carry, irrespective to a point of the level of sales achieved. The net profit is worked out by:

  Total gross margin minus overheads = net profit

Wherever possible, the overheads should be based on existing data, but this will be difficult for a new business. In this case, realistic figures for the different expenses can be obtained or calculated from a number of sources. The major items of overhead expenses, and how they can be estimated, are likely to be:

❑ Labour – calculation based on the number of staff and their pay levels. Allow for employers' National Insurance contributions as well, which amount to about 6% of the wages on average.

❏ Rates – by enquiring to the local authority. If the property is for sale or rent, the agent/landlord should be able to give an indication.
❏ Water and electricity – an estimate based on experience or from a similar business.
❏ Property repairs – a reasonable allowance for maintenance and repairs.
❏ Building depreciation – based on the cost of any investments that have been, or will be, made. The straight line basis of calculation should be used.
❏ Vehicle expenses – fuel (based on estimated mileage), repairs, servicing and MOT, insurance (quotation from a broker) and road tax.
❏ Vehicle depreciation – based on the value of vehicles or machinery.
❏ Office expenses – an allowance to cover telephone, stationery, postage, etc.
❏ Marketing – the cost of placing adverts, producing and distributing fliers, etc.
❏ Insurance – quotation from an insurance company for the appropriate cover. This may include employers' liability, public liability, premises, and loss through fire or theft.
❏ Fees – the costs of an accountant, plus possibly solicitors, consultants and any other professional advisers.
❏ Other – to allow for the inevitable unexpected!
❏ Rent – from the landlord/agent, or the rent offered for the premises.
❏ Bank interest and charges – the bank should be able to provide details on the costs of running a business account and of repaying any loans. Interest on an overdraft is more difficult to estimate at this point and is often best left until a cash flow forecast has been prepared.

Additional guidance can be found in the *Equine Business Guide*, published by Warwickshire College and the Welsh Institute of Rural Studies.

The completed budget from the example above, to illustrate the layout, is shown below.

		£
Gross margins		
Full liveries	10 @ £2,500	25,000
Dealing horses	8 @ £860	6,880
Teaching 5 hours/week	@ £12	3,000
Total gross margin		**34,880**
Overhead expenses		
Labour		13,000
Rates and water		2,600
Machinery expenses		5,200
Other		6,000
		26,800
Net profit		**8,080**

A full example of gross margin budgets and a system budget is given in the

Case Study later in this chapter. The assumptions behind the figures in a budget are often important, and the example shows how these can be explained.

Consider alternatives

It may be that slight variations on the budgeted plan could be more profitable. For example, including more of a lower gross margin enterprise may allow overhead expenses to be reduced by more than the loss of gross margin. Before deciding on the final plan, these possibilities should be considered.

Budgets for an existing business

The process is very similar to that outlined above, but with the advantage of having data of previous performance on which to base the budgets. A system budget should first be prepared for the current position, to show the profit that could be made. The profitability of any alternatives can than be compared to this figure, to see whether any changes are worth pursuing.

Benefits of the gross margin/system budget

This approach to budgeting a business has a number of advantages:

- ❑ Enterprise gross margins show which activities are most likely to be profitable.
- ❑ Having prepared a budget, it is easy to calculate the effect of changing the combination of enterprises, especially if a computer spreadsheet has been used.
- ❑ Similarly, changes in performance levels of the enterprises can be evaluated.

Case Study

To assess whether her ideas could work, Linda prepared the following budgets. These look at the expected position in year two when the business is operating at a normal level. The main assumptions in the budgets are explained as notes.

Gross margins

School ponies	**£/pony**
Sales	
Lessons (a)	5,090
Variable costs	
Replacement cost (b)	150
Concentrate feed (c)	142
Hay (d)	117
Straw (e)	78
Farrier	160
Veterinary and medicines	90
Grassland expenses	15
	752
Gross margin per pony	**4,338**

Notes
(a) Lessons charged at £6.50 per half hour (£5.53 excluding VAT), average use 10 hours per week, over 46 weeks per year to allow for holidays and injury.
(b) Ponies bought for £1,200, kept for six years and sold for £300.
(c) Stabled in barn for six months, fed 3 kg per day, cost £260 per tonne.
(d) 1.5 bales per week when stabled, cost £3 per bale.
(e) Two bales per week when stabled, cost £1.50 per bale.

School horses	**£/horse**
Sales	
Lessons (a)	6,577
Variable costs	
Replacement cost (b)	266
Concentrate feed (c)	568
Hay (d)	390
Straw (e)	234
Farrier	240
Veterinary and medicines	120
Grassland expenses	15
	1,833
Gross margin per horse	**4,744**

Notes
(a) Lessons average £12 per hour (£10.21 excluding VAT), average use 14 hours per week, 46 weeks per year.
(b) Horses bought for £2,400, kept for six years and sold for £800.
(c) Fed 6 kg per day, cost £260 per tonne.
(d) 2.5 bales per week, cost £3 per bale.
(e) Three bales per week, cost £1.50 per bale.

Full livery horses	**£/horse**
Sales	
Livery fees (a)	2,872
Sundry income (b)	250
	3,122
Variable costs	
Concentrate feed (c)	490
Hay (d)	338
Straw (e)	203
Grassland expenses	15
	1,046
Gross margin per horse	**2,076**

Notes
(a) Livery fee £75 (£63.83 excluding VAT), occupancy for 45 weeks.
(b) Income from lessons, clipping and transport services.
(c) Fed 6 kg per day, cost £260 per tonne.
(d) 2.5 bales per week, cost £3 per bale.
(e) Three bales per week, cost £1.50 per bale.

Grassland expenses (10 acres)	**£**
Fertiliser	150
Fertiliser application	50
Topping	75
Chain harrowing	50
	325
Cost per horse or pony	**15**

Notes:
(a) Wages	£/week
Assistant head girl	130
Grooms	80
Working pupil	40
Weekend helper	30

Annual labour cost £27,040, plus £1,622 for employers' National Insurance contributions.
(b) £200 per month, to cover tax, insurance, fuel, maintenance and repairs.
(c) Insurance of tack, horses and stables; employers' liability and public liability.

System budget	£
Gross margins	
School ponies 6 @ £4,338	26,026
School horses 8 @ £4,744	37,950
Livery horses 8 @ £2,076	16,609
Total gross margin	**80,585**
Overhead expenses	
Wages and NI (a)	28,662
Rent	8,000
Rates	3,000
Water	600
Electricity	600
Vehicle expenses (b)	2,400
Vehicle depreciation £8,000 @ 25%	2,000
Property repairs and maintenance	2,000
Buildings depreciation £20,000 @ 4%	800
Tack repairs and replacement	1,000
Insurance (c)	2,500
Advertising	800
Telephone, office expenses and fees	2,000
Loan interest £20,000 @ 14%	2,800
Bank interest and charges	2,000
	59,162
Net profit	**21,423**
To cover:	
Private drawings	£8,000
Loan repayments	£4,000

These figures show that the business is capable of generating enough profit to cover the private drawings and loan repayments.

Exercise

A livery yard is considering expanding by building some new stables and an outdoor manege. The manager wants to know whether this will make the business more profitable.

Without any changes, the expected position for the next year is:

Per horse	Sales	Variable costs
	£	£
7 Full livery horses	3,000	800
5 DIY liveries	1,000	200
6 dealing horses	3,200	250 plus purchase price 1,800

Overhead expenses are expected to be:

	£
Labour	9,000
Rates	1,800
Other	8,000

Prepare:
(1) Gross margin budgets for each of the three enterprises.
(2) A system budget to show the expected net profit.

The proposed expansion will allow prices of full and DIY liveries to be increased, as well as more horses to be taken. The new position will be:

12 Full livery horses	Sales £3,250 per horse
8 DIY liveries	Sales £1,100 per horse

The dealing side of the business will be unchanged, but a new activity of a breaking and schooling livery will be introduced. This is expected to attract 12 horses per year, with sales of £540 and variable costs of £100 per horse.
  Extra overhead expenses will be:

	£
Labour	6,000
Building depreciation	2,000
Rates	2,000
Interest on loan	4,000
Other	3,000

Prepare:
(1) Revised gross margin budgets for the three enterprises.
(2) A system budget to show the expected net profit of the new system.

Appendix: Gross Margins of Other Enterprises

These gross margins are included as a guide to content, as each situation will require its own figures. Further guidance can be found in the *Equine Business Guide*.

Brood mare	£
Sales	
Sale of 2-year-old	2,000
Variable costs	
Mare replacement cost*	100
Feed	300
Hay	180
Bedding	150
Veterinary and farrier	150
Stud fee	200
Livery fee at stud	150
Grazing costs	70
	1,300
Gross margin per mare	**700**

*This is the cost to maintain the breeding herd. If it is assumed that a mare can be bought for £1,500, bred from for eight years and sold for £700, then this gives the replacement cost of £100/year, i.e.

£1,500 – 700 = <u>£800</u> = £100/year
          8 years

Stallion at stud	£
Sales	
Stud fees 25 @ £200	5,000
Mares' livery 25 @ £20/week for 4 weeks	2,000
	7,000
Variable costs	
Replacement cost*	1,000
Feed	300
Hay	180
Bedding	150
Veterinary and farrier	150
	1,780
Gross margin per stallion	**5,220**

*This will not be needed if the stallion is leased or on loan. Instead, any associated costs would be entered.

Trekking	£
Sales	
Trekking income 100 days @ £25	2,500
Variable costs	
Replacement cost	100
Feed	60
Hay	80
Bedding	50
Veterinary and farrier	150
Grazing costs	30
	470
Gross margin per mount	**2,030**

Race training	£
Sales	
Training fees @ £200/week*	8,000
Variable costs	
Feed	400
Hay	200
Bedding	150
Grazing costs	30
	780
Gross margin per horse	**7,220**

*Fee varies greatly with the type of training (flat, National Hunt, point-to-point) and reputation of the yard and trainer.

Retailing (feed, tack or tuck sales)	£
Sales	5,000
Variable costs	
Stock purchases	3,000
Other costs – e.g. haulage	—
Gross margin	**2,000**

The gross margin will depend on the mark-up charged on sales, e.g. buy for £10, sell for £15; the mark-up is £5, or 50%. Typical rates of mark-up are:

Feed	10–20%
Tack	50–100%
Tuck – chocolates and sweets	25–30%
– drinks	40–60%

A large yard may justify having vending machines, which are usually supplied by the distributor in return for a percentage (15–20%) of sales.

Shows and competitions	£
Sales	
Entries 30 @ £5	150
Sponsorship	20
Trade stands	—
Advertising	—
Parking and programme sales	—
	170
Variable costs	
Prize money	30
Rosettes	10
Judges' expenses	10
Facility hire (toilets, PA system, jumps, etc.)	—
Publicity, programmes	—
Affiliation fees, score sheets	—
	50
Gross margin	**120**

The figures will vary greatly depending on the scale of the competition. The above is for a small unaffiliated dressage or show jumping contest. A three day event will be much more complex.

Facility hire; freelance teaching

These do not fit into the gross margin format, as they tend to just bring in income and have no obvious variable costs. Income from these sources can be shown in the budgets as:

Freelance teaching 4 hours/week @ £15	3,000
Arena hire 1 hour/week @ £5	250

Chapter 9
What About Next Year?
Forecasting Profit

A budget to forecast the profit for a particular year is basically a projected trading and profit and loss account (TP&L a/c for short). It is therefore presented in the same layout. Such a budget can give confidence to the bank manager, and provide a guideline and budget target for the business owner.

The budget will need to include the effects of any changes planned during the year, and possibly changes in stock levels. Most of the figures will also appear in the cash flow forecast, which is the subject of the next chapter. Some people prefer to prepare the cash flow first, and then the profit.

Five stages are involved in preparing the profit forecast. These will be illustrated with reference to the budgeting situation used as an example in the previous chapter.

Opening Stock Position

How many horses does the business own at the start of the year? What other stocks does it have? Staying with the example from chapter 8, the manager wants to prepare a profit forecast for the year commencing 1 October 199_. On this date the business will own:

	£
One dealing horse valued at	2,200
Feed and bedding stocks	500
Opening stock value of	2,700

Planned Position for Closing Stock at the End of the Year

The example business intends to have:

	£
Two dealing horses worth	4,500
Feed and bedding stocks	500
Closing stock	5,000

Expected Sales for the Year

The gross margin budgets prepared in the previous chapter can be helpful, and these should be referenced to see how the figures below have been worked out. At this stage, due allowance should be made for any changes that will be taking place in the business.

The livery side of the example business is not yet at full capacity, with only eight of the ten stables filled. However the manager expects to fill these during the course of the coming year. The gross margin budget is:

	£
Sales	
Livery fees	3,250
Direct costs	
Feed	400
Hay	200
Bedding	150
	750
Gross margin per livery	**2,500**

Using these figures, the estimate of livery income is:

	£
Eight horses for the whole year @ £3,250	26,000
Two horses for part of the year @ say £1,600	3,200
	29,200

In a similar way, the income from dealing can be estimated as:

Eight horses @ £3,200	25,600

Payments for the Year

The idea here is the same as for receipts, but some of the calculations are more complex. For example, feed:

	£
Livery horses	
Eight horses for the whole year @ £400	3,200
Two horses for part of the year @ say £200	400
dealing horses eight @ £60	480
Total feed costs	4,080

The other variable costs totals can be calculated in this way, by reference to the gross margins.

Another cost to consider will be purchase of dealing horses. The business will need to buy in nine horses:

Horses sold	8	
Add horses in closing stock	+2	
Less horses in opening stock	−1	
Horses to buy	9	@ £2,000
	= £18,000	

i.e. allowance has to be made in the closing stock for buying the extra horse.

The overhead expenses are likely to be the same as those included in the system budget, unless there are any obvious reasons for a difference.

Layout of the Budget

Having worked out the figures to include in the budget, they need to be presented in the format of a TP&L a/c. This can be illustrated by the completed budget for the example, shown below.

Profit forecast for the year commencing 1 October 199_

	£	£
Sales		
Livery fees		29,200
Horses		25,600
Teaching		3,000
		57,800
Less cost of sales		
Opening stock	2,700	
Horses	18,000	
Feed	4,080	
Hay	2,200	
Bedding	1,590	
Veterinary and farrier	640	
Marketing	960	
	30,170	
Less closing stock	(5,000)	
		25,170
Gross profit		**32,630**
Overheads		
Labour		13,000
Rates and water		2,600
Machinery expenses		5,200
Other		6,000
Interest charges*		500
		27,300
Net profit		**5,330**

*The best way to estimate interest charges is to prepare a cash flow forecast.

The following have not been mentioned in the budget. They should be listed as a note underneath:

- ❏   capital items – any investments or loan repayments
- ❏   private drawings or capital introduced.

Monthly Profit Forecast

A development from preparing an annual profit forecast is to split the figures between the twelve months. These figures can then be used to monitor the progress of sales and purchases over the year. The layout is very similar, but with additional columns for each month, as well as the annual total. A further refinement is to have two columns for each month; one for the budget figures and the other for the actual result.

Case Study

Having worked out that her business ideas looked good, Linda needed to prepare profit forecasts for her first two years of trading.

Profit forecast for the year commencing 1 April 1994

Notes
(a) To allow for developments and trade to build up, assumes 32 weeks' income.
(b) Assumes full occupancy of four boxes with existing clients, 50% occupancy of remaining four stables.
(c) Six ponies @ £1,200 each; eight horses @ £2,400 each.
(d) Keep of school horses and ponies for 12 months, four liveries for whole year and four for half of year.
(e) Value of horses and ponies.
(f) Three grooms employed, instead of four.

With the sales in year 1 below the expected normal level, the business is expected to make a small loss.

	£	£
Sales		
Riding lessons (a)	57,845	
Livery fees (b)	17,362	
Sundry livery income	1,200	
		76,407
Less cost of sales		
Opening stock	0	
Horses and ponies (c)	26,400	
Concentrate feed (d)	8,090	
Hay (d)	5,664	
Straw (d)	3,441	
Farrier	2,880	
Veterinary and medicines	1,500	
Grassland expenses	325	
	48,300	
Less closing stock (e)	(23,367)	
		24,933
Gross profit		**51,474**
Overheads		
Wages and NI (f)		24,253
Rent		8,000
Rates		3,000
Water		600
Electricity		600
Vehicle expenses		2,400
Vehicle depreciation £8,000 @ 25%		2,000
Property repairs and maintenance		2,000
Buildings depreciation £20,000 @ 4%		800
Tack repairs and replacement		1,000
Insurance		2,500
Advertising		800
Telephone, office expenses and fees		2,000
Loan interest £20,000 @ 14%		2,800
Bank interest (from cash flow)		2,214
		54,967
Net profit (loss)		**(3,493)**
Capital expenses – building works		£20,000
– loan repayments		£4,000
– tack for 14 mounts		£4,500
Private drawings		£8,000

Profit forecast for the year commencing 1 April 1995

	£	£
Sales		
Riding lessons	83,152	
Livery fees	22,979	
Sundry livery income	2,000	
		108,131
Less cost of sales		
Opening stock	23,367	
Concentrate feed	9,325	
Hay	6,522	
Straw	3,960	
Farrier	2,880	
Veterinary and medicines	1,500	
Grassland expenses	325	
	47,879	
Less closing stock	(20,333)	
		27,546
Gross profit		**80,585**
Overheads		
Wages and NI		28,662
Rent		8,000
Rates		3,000
Water		600
Electricity		600
Vehicle expenses		2,400
Vehicle depreciation £6,000 @ 25%		1,500
Property repairs and maintenance		2,000
Buildings depreciation £20,000 @ 4%		800
Tack repairs and replacement		1,000
Insurance		2,500
Advertising		800
Telephone, office expenses and fees		2,000
Loan interest £20,000 @ 14%		2,240
Bank interest (from cash flow)		1,565
		57,667
Net profit		**22,918**

For the second year, all sales and costs are assumed to be for operating at the normal level of trade.

Capital expenses – loan repayments	£4,000
Private drawings	£9,000

Comments
With a high level of initial expenditure and reduced income, a small loss in the first year is to be expected. The second year looks much more healthy

with the profit sufficient to leave a surplus after covering loan repayments and private drawings.

Exercise

Refer back to the exercise in the previous chapter. Prepare a profit forecast for the year commencing in January. This will include the proposed expansion, so at the start of the year there will be seven full liveries and five DIY liveries. These numbers will increase during the year to twelve full liveries and eight DIY liveries
Assume that:

(1) Increased prices from horses already on the yard will be received for the whole year.

(2) Income from the extra horses will be half of that for a full year.

(3) Opening stock is one horse, plus feed, etc. worth £3,000. The closing stock figure will be the same.

(4) The extra labour cost in the year will be £3,000, rather than the £6,000 for a full year.

(5) All of the other extra overhead expenses will have to be paid in full.

Use the following layout:

Profit forecast for the year commencing 1 January 199_

Sales
Full livery fees
DIY livery fees
Horses

Less cost of sales
Opening stock
Horses
Variable costs

Less closing stock

Gross profit

Overheads
Labour
Rates
Building depreciation
Interest on loan
Other

Net profit

Chapter 10
Will the Bank Balance Balance?
The Cash Flow Forecast

The cash flow forecast is the most important and useful budget, both for the manager and any lenders of finance. Its main uses are:

❑ To identify the timing and size of any borrowing requirement.
❑ In support of a request to the bank for any funding needed. It will show how much money is required, and that it can be repaid at the due time.
❑ To plan the timing of sales and payments, to try and control the size of the overdraft needed. This might involve delaying expenses, particularly large capital sums, until the business has more money. Alternatively the business might seek to bring forward sales.
❑ For budgetary control purposes. By monitoring the actual figures as the year progresses against those in the budget, problems can quickly be spotted and appropriate action taken. This topic is covered in detail in chapter 12.
❑ To provide the most reliable evidence on whether business proposals are viable. If the business will not be generating a cash surplus after two years then the ideas should probably be placed on the scrap heap.

Preparing the Cash Flow Forecast

The usual layout for a cash flow forecast is illustrated in Figure 10.1, with some example figures entered. A number of stages are involved in preparation of the forecast.

Data to include

Any movements of cash through the business bank account must be included, whether they are of a trading, capital or private nature. These then need to be allocated to the month in which the money will be either paid or received.

The profit forecast, prepared in the previous chapter, will provide most of the figures, although several points need to be borne in mind:

(1) Leave out of the cash flow forecast any items from the profit forecast that *do not* involve an actual cash movement. The main items here are depreciation and stock valuations.

Cash flow forecast for the year commencing April 199_

	April	May	June	July	...	Total
Receipts						
Stud fees	2,000	4,000	4,000	3,000	...	
Youngstock	0	0	0	7,000	...	
Total	2,000	4,000	4,000	10,000	...	
Payments						
Feed	400	300	200	200	...	
Bedding	250	250	0	0	...	
Veterinary	180	200	200	200	...	
Labour	1,000	1,000	1,000	750	...	
Vehicle expenses	200	200	200	200	...	
Admin expenses	250	250	250	250	...	
Private and tax	750	750	750	750	...	
Total	3,030	2,950	2,600	2,350	...	
Net cash flow	−1,030	1,050	1,400	7,650		
Opening bank	−3,000	−4,030	−2,980	−1,580	...	
Closing bank	−4,030	−2,980	−1,580	6,070	...	

Figure 10.1   Cash flow forecast layout

(2) Remember to include any other items that *do* involve movement of money. These may be:
   ❏ capital items such as investment in new buildings or vehicles, sale of assets, or loan repayments;
   ❏ private sums, such as the drawings of the owner, tax payments, or private money introduced into the business.

(3) Usually the annual total for items will be the same in the cash flow and profit forecasts. This basically assumes that there are no outstanding sums of money at either end of the year. If this is not the case, a slight adjustment for changes in debtors or creditors will have to be made. For example, in a stud business a client has not paid £300 for a stud fee, and so at the start of the year is a debtor for £300. In the coming year income from stud fees is expected to be £10,000. The total for stud fees to be included in the cash flow forecast would be £10,300, assuming that the £300 will be collected.

   Similarly, a business has built up a debt of £1,000 with the feed merchant, and intends to pay the creditor off over the next year. The total for feed in the cash flow would be the figure for next year's feed (say £8,000), plus the £1,000 debt, making £9,000 total.

(4) If the business is VAT registered, all income and costs should be entered net of VAT.

Timing of receipts and payments

Having prepared the figures that need to be included in the forecast, the next task is to decide in which month the money will be received or paid. This might not be the same month as the one in which services are provided or goods purchased.

❑ Some items will occur in each month but vary with the seasons, such as livery income and feed purchased.
❑ Others will only arise at certain times of the year, for example stud charges or hunter livery fees.
❑ Costs such as electricity, water, rates and telephone will be payable in a regular pattern, but only in certain months.
❑ Other overhead costs may be difficult to predict, or be very similar from month to month, in which case the same figure can be entered for each month. Examples of such costs may be property repairs, vehicle expenses and perhaps labour.

VAT details

Two stages now remain until the cash flow is completed. Both of these are simpler with a computer spreadsheet, as a number of calculations are involved.

If the business is VAT registered, VAT details need to be added to the figures. Receipts and payments should be entered in the cash flow exclusive of VAT, with the VAT on separate lines. The example from above is continued in Figure 10.2, with VAT details entered.

Cash flow forecast for the year commencing April 199_

	April	May	June	July	...
Receipts					
Stud fees	2,000	4,000	4,000	3,000	...
Youngstock	0	0	0	7,000	...
VAT on sales	350	700	700	1,750	...
Total	2,350	4,700	4,700	11,750	...
Payments					
Feed	400	300	200	200	...
Bedding	250	250	0	0	...
Veterinary	180	200	200	200	...
Labour	1,000	1,000	1,000	750	...
Vehicle expenses	200	200	200	200	...
Admin expenses	250	250	250	250	...
Private and tax	750	750	750	750	...
VAT on inputs	110	114	114	114	...
VAT to C&E	0	0	1,412	0	...
Total	3,140	3,064	4,126	2,464	...

Figure 10.2　Cash flow forecast with VAT details and receipts and payments totals

In the receipts section a line for 'VAT on sales' is added, in which any VAT to be received in the month is entered. Similarly, a line for 'VAT on inputs' is included in the payments section. Any VAT payable to the Customs and Excise needs to be calculated and entered in the forecast in the 'VAT to C&E' line.

For the example above, VAT would be received on stud fees and youngstock sales. Hence, VAT on sales for April is:

£2,000 × 17.5% (the current VAT rate) = £350.

It would be paid on veterinary, vehicle and administration expenses.

The VAT to C&E line is worked out on the assumption, which is usual for horse businesses, that VAT returns are completed quarterly. The procedure is to total the figures for VAT on sales and VAT on inputs for the quarter. The difference between these is the sum that is owed to Customs and Excise, and this is entered in the last month of the quarter.

	VAT on sales £	VAT on inputs £
April	350	110
May	700	114
June	700	114
	1,750	338
Difference payable to C&E £1,412		

Interest charges and closing bank balance

To complete the cash flow, the bank balance, month by month, and any interest charges need to be worked out. The completed cash flow example is shown in Figure 10.3. This shows that the business needs an overdraft facility of £4,000 to cover the peak in April.

The following calculations are involved:

(1) Interest needs to be charged only if the opening bank balance is negative. In reality, interest on a bank overdraft is calculated daily on the closing balance, but the formula gives a sufficiently accurate estimate. If the opening bank balance is positive, there is no interest. If it is negative (minus):

$$\text{Interest} = \frac{\text{overdrawn bank balance} \times \text{interest rate } \%}{12}$$

Dividing the annual interest rate by 12 gives the interest charge for one month. So for April, the calculation is:

$$\text{Interest} = \frac{£3,000 \times 12\%}{12} = £30$$

Cash flow forecast for the year commencing April 199_				
	April	**May**	**June**	**July**	...

Receipts					
Stud fees	2,000	4,000	4,000	3,000	...
Youngstock	0	0	0	7,000	...
VAT on sales	350	700	700	1,750	...
Total	2,350	4,700	4,700	11,750	...
Payments					
Feed	400	300	200	200	...
Bedding	250	250	0	0	...
Veterinary	180	200	200	200	...
Labour	1,000	1,000	1,000	750	...
Vehicle expenses	200	200	200	200	...
Admin expenses	250	250	250	250	...
Private and tax	750	750	750	750	...
Interest @ 12%	30	38	22	17	
VAT on inputs	110	114	114	114	...
VAT to C&E	0	0	1,412	0	...
Total	3,170	3,102	4,148	2,481	...
Net cash flow	–820	1,598	552	9,269	...
Opening bank	–3,000	–3,820	–2,222	–1,670	...
Closing bank	–3,820	–2,222	–1,670	–7,599	...

Figure 10.3 Cash flow forecast with interest and bank balance calculated

(2) Net cash flow is the difference between receipts and payments for each month.

Net cash flow = total receipts minus total payments

(3) Opening bank (balance) in the first month is the bank balance at the start of the forecast. For later months it is the closing balance from the previous month.

(4) Closing bank (balance) is the expected bank balance at the end of each month. It is useful for estimating the size of any overdraft needed, or identifying times in the year when there may be surplus cash.

Closing bank = net cash flow plus opening bank

All of these calculations need to be made for each month. Use of a computer spreadsheet reduces the chance of errors creeping in, as well as being much quicker. A further advantage is that if a number is changed, the figures will recalculate automatically, saving the laborious task of working them all out again manually.

Case Study

Linda prepared the cash flow forecasts shown in Figures 10.4 and 10.5 to include in her business plan.

The first year (1994/95) forecast showed that her overdraft would peak in May at nearly £26,000. After this it dropped to a level of around £20,000 for the remainder of the year. These figures informed her that she would need an overdraft facility of £26,000, as well as the £20,000 loan taken out in April.

The cash flow for 1995/96 gave her a lot of confidence that the business would be a success, with the overdraft reduced to £5,000 by the end of the year.

	Apr	May	June	July	Aug	Sept	Oct	Nov	Dec	Jan	Feb	Mar	Total
Receipts													
Riding lessons			4,627	5,784	6,942	6,942	6,942	5,784	4,628	4,628	5,784	5,784	57,845
Livery fees	964	964	964	964	1,203	1,203	1,850	1,850	1,850	1,850	1,850	1,850	17,362
Sundry livery	80	80	80	80	100	100	100	100	120	120	120	120	1,200
Loan	20,000												20,000
VAT on sales	183	183	992	1,195	1,443	1,443	1,556	1,353	1,155	1,155	1,357	1,357	13,371
Total receipts	21,227	1,227	6,663	8,023	9,688	9,688	10,448	9,087	7,753	7,753	9,111	9,111	109,778
Payments													
Horses/ponies	13,200	13,200											26,400
Concentrate feed	250	560	560	560	620	620	780	780	780	860	860	860	8,090
Hay	122	354	354	354	460	460	540	540	620	620	620	620	5,664
Straw	1,000					2,440							3,440
Farrier, veterinary and medicines		260	412	412	412	412	412	412	412	412	412	412	4,380
Grassland expenses			200		125								325
Wages and NI	2,020	2,021	2,021	2,021	2,021	2,021	2,021	2,021	2,021	2,021	2,021	2,023	24,253
Rent	4000						4,000						8,000
Rates	300	300	300	300	300	300	300	300	300	300			3,000
Water	300						300						600
Electricity	150			150			150			150			600
Vehicle expenses	700	200	300	100	100	100	100	200	300	100	100	100	2,400
Property repairs	163	167	167	167	167	167	167	167	167	167	167	168	2,000
Tack	2,250	2,250	100	100	100	100	100	100	100	100	100	100	5,500
Insurance	1,250			1,250									2,500
Advertising	200	200	200	100			100						800
Telephone, etc.	500			500			500			500			2,000
Loan interest			700			700			700			700	2,800
Loan repayment												4,000	4,000
Buildings	10,000	10,000											20,000
Private drawings	666	666	666	666	666	666	666	666	668	668	668	668	8,000
Interest @12%	0	0	260	257	250	207	228	230	196	216	203	166	2,214
VAT on inputs	589	601	287	322	249	227	360	255	255	357	269	270	4,042
VAT to C&E			-119			3,282			3,193			2,973	9,329
Total payments	37,660	30,779	6,408	7,259	5,470	11,703	10,724	5,672	9,713	6,471	5,420	13,060	150,338
Net cash flow	-16,433	-29,553	256	764	4,218	-2,015	-276	3,416	-1,960	1,282	3,691	-3,949	-40,560
Opening bank	20,000	3,567	-25,986	-25,730	-24,966	-20,748	-22,763	-23,039	-19,623	-21,584	-20,302	-16,611	20,000
Closing bank	3,567	-25,986	-25,730	-24,966	-20,748	-22,763	-23,039	-19,623	-21,584	-20,302	-16,611	-20,560	-20,560

Figure 10.4   Cash flow forecast – Oxhill Stables 1994/5

	Apr	May	June	July	Aug	Sept	Oct	Nov	Dec	Jan	Feb	Mar	Total
Receipts													
Riding lessons	6,930	7,623	7,623	7,623	8,316	7,623	6,930	5,544	6,930	5,540	5,540	6,930	83,152
Livery fees	1,915	1,915	1,819	1,819	1,819	1,819	1,915	1,918	2,010	2,010	2,010	2,010	22,979
Sundry livery	120	120	120	120	120	140	210	210	210	210	210	210	2,000
VAT on sales	1,569	1,690	1,673	1,673	1,795	1,677	1,585	1,343	1,601	1,358	1,358	1,601	18,923
Total receipts	10,534	11,348	11,235	11,235	12,050	11,259	10,640	9,015	10,751	9,118	9,118	10,751	127,054
Payments													
Horses/ponies													0
Concentrate feed	736	710	710	710	710	710	840	840	840	840	840	840	9,326
Hay	500	500	500	500	500	500	587	587	587	587	587	587	6,522
Straw	1800					2,160							3,960
Farrier, veterinary and medicines	365	365	365	365	365	365	365	365	365	365	365	365	4,380
Grassland expenses			200		125								325
Wages and NI	2,388	2,388	2,388	2,388	2,388	2,388	2,389	2,389	2,389	2,389	2,389	2,389	28,662
Rent	4,000						4,000						8,000
Rates	300	300	300	300	300	300	300	300	300	300			3,000
Water	300						300						600
Electricity	150			150			150			150			600
Vehicle expenses	700	200	300	100	100	100	100	200	300	100	100	100	2,400
Property repairs	163	167	167	167	167	167	167	167	167	167	167	167	2,000
Tack	83	83	83	83	83	83	83	83	83	83	83	87	1,000
Insurance	1,250			1,250									2,500
Advertising	50	50	50	150	50	50	150	50	50	50	50	50	800
Telephone, etc.	500			500			500			500			2,000
Loan interest		560				560			560			560	2,240
Loan repayment												4,000	4,000
Private drawings	750	750	750	750	750	750	750	750	750	750	750	750	9,000
Interest @12%	206	246	192	189	157	96	111	116	87	83	59	24	1,565
VAT on inputs	332	241	276	346	263	241	368	263	263	351	263	264	3,470
VAT to C&E		4,084			4,296				3,633			3,439	15,453
Total payments	14,573	6,000	10,925	7,948	5,957	12,765	11,160	6,110	10,375	6,715	5,653	13,622	111,803
Net cash flow	-4,039	5,349	310	3,287	6,093	-1,506	-520	2,904	377	2,403	3,465	-2,871	15,251
Opening bank	-20,560	-24,599	-19,250	-18,940	-15,653	-9,560	-11,067	-11,587	-8,683	-8,306	-5,903	-2,438	
Closing bank	-24,599	-19,250	-18,940	-15,653	-9,560	-11,067	-11,587	-8,683	-8,306	-5,903	-2,438	-5,309	

Figure 10.5 Cash flow forecast – Oxhill Stables 1995/6

Exercise

A riding school needs to prepare a cash flow forecast for the next six months. Expected receipts and payments are:

Receipts

Jan	Feb	Mar	Apr	May	June
£1,200	£900	£1,100	£1,400	£1,400	£1,300

In addition, VAT will be charged at 17.5%.

Payments

Horses	£4,000 in March
Feed & bedding	£400/month for Jan-Apr, £200 in May and June
Labour	£400/month Jan-Mar, £500/month Apr-June
Rates	£1,000 in Apr
Other	£300/month

VAT will be paid at 17.5% only on 'Other'.

VAT returns are due in March and June.
Bank balance on 1 January is £1,500.
Interest on the overdraft is charged monthly at an annual rate of 10%.

(1) Prepare the cash flow forecast for the six months.

(2) Suggest the size of overdraft that should be requested.

Chapter 11
Completing the Picture
Capital and Cash

The profit and cash flow forecasts covered in the previous two chapters are vital for any business wishing to plan its development. To give a complete picture of the planned finances of the business, two further aspects can be covered. These are the projected balance sheet, and a reconciliation of forecast profit and cash flow.

Reconciliation of Forecast Profit and Cash Flow

This explains why there may be a difference between the budgeted profit and net cash flow for the year. It is closely related to the cash flow statement (different to a cash flow forecast), which is discussed in detail in chapter 17, and it may help to read this chapter before continuing.

The purposes of the reconciliation are:

❏ to provide a mathematical check that no errors have been made when preparing the profit and cash flow forecasts;
❏ it can be used to estimate a closing bank balance for the year, if a cash flow forecast has not been prepared.

It is based on adding or subtracting various items from the forecast profit:

Forecast net profit (or loss)

+ Depreciation
+ Loans taken out
+ Capital/cash introduced
+ Capital sales
+ Decrease in stocks (or – Increase in stocks)
+ Decrease in debtors (or – Increase in debtors)
+ Increase in creditors (or – Decrease in creditors)

– Loan repayments
– Private drawings and tax
– Capital investments

= Net cash flow for the year

This answer should be the same as:

Closing bank balance minus opening bank balance

The reasons why different items are added to net profit while others are subtracted are discussed in chapter 17. It is unlikely that all of these items will be relevant: debtors and creditors will usually be unchanged over the year, and there may be no loans or capital investments.

If the calculation above does not reconcile, then there must be some discrepancy between the figures in the profit forecast and cash flow. The budgets then need to be checked until the reason is found.

Projected Balance Sheet

This will show how the value of the business is expected to change over the course of the year. It is important that proposals will result in the capital worth of the business increasing.

The information needs to be collected from various parts of the budgets, for example the closing bank balance from the cash flow. It then needs to be presented in the balance sheet format described in chapter 4.

Case Study

To complete the financial details in her business plan, Linda prepared the following statements.

Reconciliation of profit and cash flow forecasts for the year commencing 1/4/94

	£
Net profit (loss)	(3,493)
+ Depreciation	2,800
+ Loans taken out	20,000
– Increase in stocks	(23,367)
– Loan repayments	(4,000)
– Private drawings	(8,000)
– Capital investments	(24,500)
= **Net cash flow for the year**	**(40,560)**
From cash flow forecast:	
Opening bank balance	20,000
Closing bank balance	(20,560)
Net cash flow	**(40,560)**

Net cash flow = closing bank balance – opening bank balance

Notes on sources of information

Net profit	from the profit forecast.
Depreciation	from the profit forecast – overheads.
Loan taken out	note to the profit forecast, or from cash flow forecast.
Increase in stocks	difference between closing and opening stocks.
Loan repayments	from cash flow forecast.
Personal drawings	from cash flow forecast.
Capital investments	note to the profit forecast, or from cash flow forecast.

Opening and closing bank balances from cash flow forecast.

Projected balance sheets

Balance sheets on:	**1/4/95**	**1/4/94**
	£	**£**
Fixed assets		
Buildings	19,200	0
Vehicles	6,000	8,000
School horses and ponies	23,367	0
Tack and equipment	4,500	0
	53,067	8,000
Current assets		
Bank balance	0	20,000
Current liabilities		
Bank overdraft	20,560	0
Net current assets	(20,560)	20,000
Long-term liability		
Loan	16,000	0
Net capital	**16,507**	**28,000**
Financed by:		
Opening net capital	28,000	
+ Net profit	(3,493)	
– Private and tax	(8,000)	
	16,507	

Notes on sources of information

Buildings	£20,000 investment, less annual depreciation of £800.
Vehicles	Initial value of £8,000, less annual depreciation of 25% on reducing balance.
Horses and ponies	Initial cost of mounts (£26,400), less annual 'depreciation' or allowance for replacement of £150 per pony and £267 per horse (see gross margins in chapter 8).
Tack and equipment	Initial value (£4,500) maintained by repairs and renewals.
Bank balance	Closing balance from cash flow forecast.
Loan	Initial loan of £20,000, with annual capital repayments of £4,000.
Net profit	From profit forecast.
Private	From cash flow forecast.

Exercise _____

Linda also prepared:

❑ reconciliation of profit and cash flow forecasts for the year commencing 1/4/95;
❑ projected balance sheet for 31/3/96.

Referring to data in this and the previous three chapters work out these statements. The items to include are:

❑ balance sheet – the same as those in the case study section;
❑ profit/cash flow reconciliation – there are no loans taken out or investments, and the value of stock is a decrease rather than an increase.

Chapter 12
Controlling our Destiny
The Disciplines of Budgetary Control

The idea of using plans and budgets as guidelines, along which to direct the business, has already been mentioned several times. They should never be prepared to then gather dust, but to be used as management tools. Rather than sitting back and seeing what happens, it is a case of monitoring the progress of the business, and trying to control its destiny by guiding it along the desired path.

Budgetary control disciplines can be considered as either short-term or longer term.

Short-term Budgetary Control

This is usually carried out each month, and is based on comparing the budgeted cash flow figures with what actually happens. Any deviations from the budget can be quickly spotted and appropriate action taken.

To enable this, it is best to present the cash flow forecast with two columns for each month, one headed 'Budget' and the other 'Actual'. The actual figures can then be written in each month after the book-keeping routine has been completed.

An example with budget figures for January to March, and the actual results entered to February, is shown in Figure 12.1.

The situation here is that payments, overall, have been about the same as the budget, but receipts have been low, especially sales of horses. In March it is planned to invest £10,000, which in the budget the business could afford. As events have turned out, the bank account will go overdrawn if this money is invested.

The manager is now aware of a problem, and needs to decide what action to take. To help with this decision, the reasons for the discrepancies between the budget and actual figures need to be explored, a process known as variance analysis. They could be due to one of the following.

Quantity differences

These occur when the volume of sales (or purchases) is above or below the budget. In the example above, it could be that in January:

	January		February		March	
	Budget	**Actual**	**Budget**	**Actual**	**Budget**	**Actual**
Receipts						
Lessons	2,500	2,200	2,600	2,500	2,800	
Horses	6,000	3,000	3,000	2,800	3,000	
Total receipts	8,500	5,200	5,600	5,300	5,800	
Payments						
Feed, bedding	700	750	700	760	700	
Labour	400	350	400	370	400	
Rent	0	0	0	0	3,000	
Other overheads	1,200	1,420	1,200	1,040	1,200	
New horsebox	0	0	0	0	10,000	
Total payments	2,300	2,520	2,300	2,170	15,300	
Opening bank	1,200	1,180	7,400	3,860	10,700	
Closing bank	7,400	3,860	10,700	6,990	1,200	

Figure 12.1   Cash flow with budget and actual data entered

	Planned quantity	*Actual quantity*
Sales of horses	2	1
Riding lessons sold	250	220

Price differences

These are when the discrepancy is due to prices. For example, horse sales may be £200 below budget in February because the planned horse was sold, but at a lower price.

Change in the timing of sales or purchases

This will affect the budget compared to actual figures for the month, but the discrepancy should be made right later. It could affect the size of an overdraft in the short term though, and the bank manager might need to be informed of the situation. For example, the horse that was to be sold in January may have gone lame, but will be ready for sale in March instead. This will bring the horse sales figure for the three months more in line with the budget.

Debtors or creditors outstanding

It could be that the planned level of business has been achieved during the month, in terms of quantity and price. The difference is due to the fact that the money has not been received because of late payment.

Having identified the reasons for discrepancies, especially those that are unfavourable, a plan of action can be drawn up. If a business is not meeting its budget, this is likely to involve looking at ways to either increase income, or reduce spending.

Increasing income

There are no easy answers for increasing income, but a number of possibilities can be investigated:

❏ Advertising or promotional activity to try and generate more sales.
❏ Increase prices, but the business would have to be careful that this did not result in customers leaving.
❏ Credit control procedures should be tightened if the problem is due to late payment by customers, in an attempt to get outstanding accounts paid. Persistent late payers need to be sent reminders of overdue accounts, and to be personally approached (tactfully) on the subject. As a last resort, after a reasonable period of time has passed (typically three months), outstanding debtors can be taken to the small claims court in pursuit of payment. This is a reasonably cheap and simple process.

Reducing spending

Options for reducing spending are again usually not simple to implement. They include:

❏ Careful control of costs by close monitoring of feed levels, prudent use of vehicles, etc. The private drawings of the owner should also be put under scrutiny.
❏ Running down stock levels may be possible, in the short term, as a way to save money. For example, only keeping one month's supply of hay in the barn, rather than six months'.
❏ Delay buying some items. In the example considered previously, the purchase of the horse box may have to wait until more money is available. If everything is required now, perhaps payment could be delayed on some items, although there is a danger here of becoming unpopular with suppliers.
❏ Change spending plans. Capital investments are particularly vulnerable here as the business tightens its belt. They will often be deferred until more money is available.

If, at the end of the day, the budget figures cannot be met, the bank may need to be approached for additional finance. They are more likely to respond favourably to the business that has been carefully monitoring its position, than the one that has unknowingly found itself in trouble.

Longer Term Budgetary Control

This involves looking at the performance of the business over a longer period of time, usually the financial year. Variance analysis can again identify reasons for any differences between the budgeted and actual results.

It is possible to work out the effects of the quantity and price differences to help in planning the best action for the future.

Example 1
A riding school found that children's lessons were more popular than expected:

	Budget	Actual
Number of lessons per week	240	260
Average charge per lesson	£10	£9
Weekly income	£2,400	£2,340

How much of this difference is due to the number of lessons, and how much to the lower price?
Difference due to quantity (lessons):

Quantity difference × actual price
= 20 lessons x £9   = £180

Difference due to price:

Budgeted quantity x price difference
= 240 lessons × (-£1)   = –£240

Overall difference   –£60

This suggests that efforts should be made to increase prices next year.

Example 2
Feed costs. The riding school planned to use 36 tonnes of hard feed during the year, at a cost of £240 per tonne. The actual result was 38 tonnes of feed used, at an average cost of £220 per tonne.

	Budget	Actual
Total feed use (tonnes)	36	38
Feed cost per tonne	£240	£220
Total feed cost	£8,640	£8,360

This is a favourable variance in that the cost was £280 less than budgeted. The reasons for the difference are still worth exploring.
Difference due to quantity (tonnes):

Quantity difference × actual price
= 2 tonnes × £220   = £440

Difference due to price:

Budgeted quantity × price difference
= 36 tonnes × (–£20)   = –£720

Overall difference   –£280

This shows that, despite feed costs being below the budget, there is scope for further savings by more careful control of feeding.

As well as variance analysis, a detailed study of the accounts should also be carried out at the end of each year, using the techniques described in Part 3 of this book.

The information found by these investigations then needs to be used to assess how well the business is doing, and plan for the future. This may involve fine tuning of the plan, or a major rethink, thus linking budgetary control with the whole process of planning and budgeting. The flow chart in Figure 12.2 illustrates the ongoing nature of this process, as plans are amended in the light of actual results.

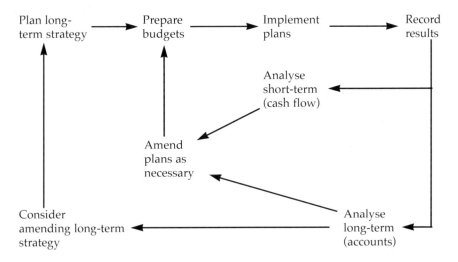

Figure 12.2   The cycle of business planning and budgetary control

Case Study

The data in Figure 12.3 has been extracted from Linda's cash analysis book in chapter 3 and her cash flow forecast for 1995/6 in chapter 10. These figures indicated that income was falling below the target. Closer examination of livery income revealed that the full livery uptake was down, partly offset by some DIY liveries:

| | April | | May | | June | |
	Budget	**Actual**	**Budget**	**Actual**	**Budget**	**Actual**
Receipts						
Lessons	6,930	6,100	7,623	5,796	7,623	
Livery	1,915	1,650	1,915	1,360	1,819	
Sundry income	120	200	120	47	120	
Total receipts	8.965	7,950	9,658	7,203	9,562	

Figure 12.3   Budget and actual figures for Oxhill Stables, April–June 1995

	Budget	Actual results	
		April	May
Weeks of full livery	30	24	20
Full livery income	£1,915	£1,530	£1,270
Weeks of DIY livery		8	6
DIY livery income		£120	£90
Total income	£1,915	£1,650	£1,360

In response to this situation, Linda advertised to attract two new full livery horses to fill the spaces that had become available. The riding school publicity was also increased to attract extra business over the summer months.

Chapter 13
The 'What If?' Situations
Partial Budgets for Simple Changes

Everyone who runs, or works in, a business is likely to get 'what if …?' ideas. It could be a new activity, or changing the way things are done. These ideas may have little or no impact on most of the existing activities. Partial budgets are a simple way to approach these 'what if?' type of situations. The aim is to see what extra annual net profit could be generated by the idea.

Suitable problems to tackle by means of a partial budget will usually fall into one of three types.

(1) Increasing one enterprise at the expense of another, such as more school horses and fewer liveries.
(2) Expanding the business, by means of increasing an enterprise or the introduction of a new one. Examples could be the construction of more stables to accommodate extra horses, buying in a youngster to school on and sell, or holding a competition.
(3) A change of technique or technology. Examples here could be installing a horse walker to enable a reduction in labour costs, or buying equipment for making hay instead of using a contractor's services.

A partial budget is laid out under four headings:

Gains   *Losses*
Extra income   Income lost
Costs saved   Extra costs
Gains minus losses = extra net profit

Depending on the situation, sometimes only two of these headings are needed.

Example:
Taking a full livery horse instead of a DIY livery

Extra income	£	*Income lost*	£
Full livery fees @ £70/week	3,500	DIY fees @ £20/week	1,000
		Extra costs	
		Feed, bedding, etc.	800
		Labour	1,000
	3,500		2,800
		Extra net profit	**700**

A key point is that the budget shows the extra *annual* net profit. Items of income and costs therefore need to be for a typical year, not the first year that the change is introduced. There are some important implications arising from this, which are illustrated in the more complex example below.

Example:
A riding school has demand for more school horses, but to accommodate them needs to build five new stables. The partial budget is shown in Figure 13.1.

			£
Extra income			
Lessons – 5 horses @ 10 hours/week @ £10 for 50 weeks			25,000
Extra costs		£	
(a) Variable costs			
Feed	5 horses @ £400	2,000	
Hay	5 horses @ £250	1,250	
Bedding	5 horses @ £150	750	
Veterinary and medicines	5 horses @ £120	600	
Farrier	5 horses @ £240	1,200	
			5,800
(b) Extra horses			
Annual replacement cost – 5 horses @ £150		750	
Interest on capital – 5 horses @ £1,500 = £7,500 @ 12%		900	
			1,650
(c) New stables			
Stables – capital cost £12,000, written off over 10 years, depreciation per year		1,200	
Interest on capital – £12,000 @ 12%		1,440	
			2,640
(d) Other overheads			
Insurance		120	
Rates		250	
Electricity, water, etc.		1,000	
Additional labour		5,000	
			6,370
Total extra costs			16,460
Extra net profit			**8,540**

Figure 13.1 Partial budget for investment in stabling to accommodate extra school horses

Key points

Depreciation

If an idea involves capital investment in buildings, machinery or fixtures, depreciation should be included in the budget, and not the initial capital cost. The depreciation should be calculated as the average annual depreciation over the life of the asset. For the example above, with stables costing £12,000, to be written off (i.e. depreciated to zero) in 10 years, the annual depreciation is:

$$\frac{£12,000}{10 \text{ years}} = £1,200 \text{ per year}$$

Another example is a horse box purchased for £15,000, and to be kept for five years, with resale value after this time of £5,000. Average annual depreciation is:

$$\frac{£15,000 - 5,000}{5 \text{ years}} = £2,000 \text{ per year}$$

A general formula is:

$$\text{Annual depreciation} = \frac{\text{Purchase price minus Sale price}}{\text{Expected life of asset}}$$

Replacement cost of horses

Where a proposal involves acquiring extra horses, the annual replacement cost should be used in the budget, and not the initial cost of buying the horses. In the example above, extra school horses cost £1,500 to buy and have a working life of six years, with value at the end expected to be £600. The annual replacement cost will be:

$$\frac{£1,500 - 600}{6 \text{ years}} = £150 \text{ per year}$$

Extra capital

An important consideration is whether additional capital (money) will be tied up in the business as a result of the proposed change. If it is, then an interest charge needs to be included in the budget.

Capital items
For capital items, this interest should be calculated on the cost of the investment. Extra horses should be treated in this way as well.

Variable costs
If a proposal will bring in a regular income, such as livery fees or lessons, then any interest on the variable costs such as feed, etc. can be ignored.

However, if money will be tied up for a significant period of time before an income is received, then this needs to be included in the interest calculation.

For example, if buying a mare to put in foal and then sell the foal as a two year old, money will be tied up for three years. Taking the costs of feed and keep for the mare (and foal to two years old) to total £1,500, and interest at 10%, the calculation will be:

£750 (half of £1,500) × 10% = £75 × 3 years = £225

£750 is used instead of £1,500 to allow for the fact that not all of the costs of keep are paid at the beginning of the three years, but gradually during this period.

Partial budgets are a simple way to assess whether an idea is likely to lead to extra profit. Having established this, it may then be necessary to use more complicated budgeting techniques, such as a cash flow forecast, especially if a large capital investment is involved.

Case Study

To complement Linda's stables business, her father is thinking of building a cross country course around the farm. The cost of construction will be £10,000, and it is expected to attract about 1,250 rounds per year at a charge of £5 each. The partial budget looks as follows.

	£	£
Extra income		
Rounds 1,250 @ £5		6,250
Extra costs		
Depreciation £10,000 over 10 years	1,000	
Maintenance and repairs	500	
Interest on £10,000 @ 12%	1,200	
		2,700
Extra profit		**3,550**

The partial budget suggests that it would be a profitable sideline to develop the course.

Exercises _____

Prepare partial budgets for the following situations:

(1) A riding school/livery yard needs four more school horses but cannot accommodate then without getting rid of four DIY liveries.

Per horse		£
School horse	– income	4,400
	– variable costs	1,200
	– purchase cost	1,800
	– sale value	1,000 (after four years)
DIY livery income		900
Interest rate		12%
Extra labour (total)		3,000

(2) A stud at present makes 10 ha (25 acres) of hay, and employs the services of a contractor to do all the work. The manager wonders whether it would be better to own the equipment instead, as they already have a large enough tractor.

	£
Contractor's charge	120/ha
Cost of machinery needed (to be bought second hand)	5,000
Estimated value after four years	1,000
Spares and repairs for machinery	250/year
Tractor running costs for hay making	200/year
Interest rate	10%

Chapter 14

If it doesn't go to Plan
Sensitivity and Break Even Analysis

What will happen if the plans, despite the best efforts of the manager, do not work out? How serious will it be if the sales are less than expected, or the costs higher? The wise manager, and lenders of finance, will want to know the answers to such questions. These are provided by the techniques of sensitivity and break even analysis.

Sensitivity Analysis

A sensitivity analysis looks at the effect of a change in a key assumption, such as price or quantity, on the outcome of a budget. It can be applied to any type of budget. An example could be a livery horse gross margin.

	£
Sales	
Livery fees 50 weeks @ £70	3,500
Variable costs	
Feed	400
Hay	250
Bedding	100
	750
Gross margin per livery	**2,750**

Sensitivity
Price +/−£5 /week, gross margin +/−£250
Uptake +/−1 week, gross margin +/−£70

If the budget is very sensitive to a small change in a key price or output, then the proposal is going to be risky: any forecast profit could be lost if the budget target is missed by only a small amount.

The idea of sensitivity analysis can be extended to whole business budgets. Figures can be worked out based on realistic expectations, and then on pessimistic assumptions. If the pessimistic budget shows the proposals to be unviable, or only marginally viable, then the venture needs to be entered upon with much more caution.

Break Even Analysis

The aim of a break even analysis is to find the level of output (or sales) where the business reaches the break even point, which is where it has covered all of its costs. Any extra sales beyond this point will start to generate a net profit. Having found the break even point, a judgement can be made on how likely it is that this level of sales can be exceeded.

An example to look at is the cross country course proposal in the previous chapter, for which the following partial budget was prepared.

	£	£
Extra income		
Rounds 1,250 @ £5		6,250
Extra costs		
Depreciation £10,000 over 10 years	1,000	
Maintenance and repairs	500	
Interest on £10,000 @ 12%	1,200	
		2,700
Extra net profit		**3,550**

The break even number of rounds will be the amount needed to cover all of the costs, i.e. £2,700. To find the break even point, divide by the charge per round:

$$\frac{£2,700}{£5} = 540 \text{ rounds per year}$$

It is very likely that this level of sales could be achieved, therefore the project stands a good chance of making a profit.

This is a straightforward calculation, because all of the costs are 'fixed' in that they are not dependent on the number of rounds. When some costs vary with the level of output the situation is more complicated, but it is easily dealt with on a graph, or break even chart.

Example: livery yard with capacity for up to 20 horses. Fixed costs are £20,000, variable costs £1,200 per livery, and income £3,000 per horse. The break even chart is shown in Figure 14.1.

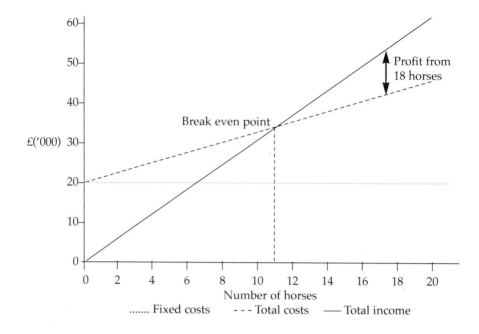

Figure 14.1   Break even chart for livery stables

Notes
(1) The total cost line is the variable costs added to the fixed costs.
(2) The break even point is where the total income equals the total costs, which from the chart can be seen to be with just over 11 horses.
(3) At a given number of horses the amount of net profit achieved is the difference between the total income and total costs. For example, the profit with 18 horses:
Income   £54,000
Total costs   £41,600
Net profit   £12,400
(4) A level of sales achieved above the break even point is called the margin of safety, i.e. the amount of sales that can be lost before the business is in a loss making situation.

Sensitivity can also be looked at on a break even chart, by showing the effects of changes in costs or income. For example, if the income per horse can be increased from £3,000 to £3,500, the modified chart is shown in Figure 14.2. The break even point is now with 9 horses, and at 18 horses the profit has increased to £21,400.

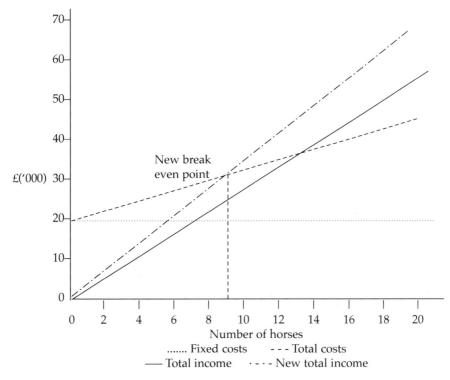

Figure 14.2 Break even chart for livery stables with increased income

---

Case Study/Exercise

Sensitivity analysis

In this section, the case study and exercise are combined, with both relating to Oxhill Stables. The answer to the first part of each exercise is given to illustrate the technique. It is based on the budgets for Oxhill Stables shown in chapter 8.

(1) Prepare sensitivity calculations for:
  (a) the school horses based on +/–£1/hour lesson price and +/–1 hour /week teaching hours;
  (b) the school ponies based on +/–£1/hour lesson price and +/–1 hour/week teaching hours;
  (c) the livery horses based on +/–£5/week (excluding VAT) livery fee and +/–1 week occupancy.

Example – answer for school horses (a)
Working from the gross margin budget:

	£/horse
Sales	
Lessons (a)	6,577
Variable costs	
Replacement cost	266
Concentrate feed	568
Hay	390
Straw	234
Farrier	240
Veterinary and medicines	120
Grassland expenses	15
	1,833
Gross margin per horse	**4,744**

Lessons average £12 per hour (£10.21 excluding VAT), average use 14 hours per week, 46 weeks per year.

Sensitivity
Lesson price +/–£1/hour (excluding VAT), gross margin +/–£644
  (£1/hour × 14 hours/week × 46 weeks = £644)
Teaching hours +/–1 hour/week, gross margin +/–£470
  (1 hour × £10.21 (ex. VAT) × 46 weeks = £470)

Exercise

Break even analysis
A riding school has fixed costs of £50,000. Annual income, from horses working 12 hours per week, is £6,000 each. Variable costs (including labour) are £2,500 per horse. The yard has capacity for 20 horses.

(1) Prepare a break even chart to find the number of horses (working 12 hours per week) at which the business will break even, and the profit with 20 horses.

(2) If the horses work 14 hours per week, income rises to £7,000. What would the break even position be in this situation?

Chapter 15
A Sound Investment?
Techniques of Investment Appraisal

The budgeting techniques described in the previous chapters show whether a proposed investment is likely to increase the profits of a business. Important questions still remain, though.

❏ Is the investment the best use of the money? Perhaps it would be better left in the bank on deposit.
❏ Two projects competing for the same money – which one should go ahead?

It is to questions such as these that the techniques of investment appraisal provide answers.

Each of the four methods described here require, first of all, that the preliminary budgeting has taken place. The size of the investment and the likely returns over the coming years are therefore known.

Pay Back Period

This is the amount of time that is taken for the returns from the investment to repay the initial sum. For example, expected costs and returns from a project costing £10,000 are shown below.

Year	Income	Costs	Net cash flow	Cumulative net cash flow
	£	£	£	£
1	4,000	2,500	1,500	1,500
2	6,000	3,000	3,000	4,500
3	6,000	3,000	3,000	7,500
4	6,000	3,000	3,000	10,500
5	6,000	3,000	3,000	13,500

Cumulative net cash flow is the total amount of cash that the project has generated to date.

By adding up the net cash flows, it can be seen that the investment of £10,000 has all been repaid by the end of the fourth year (3 years and 10 months, if the cash flow is even through the year).

A shorter pay back period is to be preferred. This suggests that less risk is involved with the project, and is especially important if conditions are likely to change in the future.

The pay back period technique has some advantages and disadvantages:

Advantages   *Disadvantages*
Simple technique   Ignores returns after the
Easily calculated   pay back period

It can be a useful way of initially screening ideas, to eliminate any that do not achieve a sufficiently quick pay back.

Annual Rate of Return

Annual rate of return looks at the return from an investment (in the form of net profit) compared to the initial capital cost. It is calculated by the formula:

$$\text{Annual rate of return} = \frac{\text{Average annual net profit}}{\text{Capital investment}} \times 100$$

Rather than looking at net cash returns, like the pay back period, here the concern is with net profit. An allowance for depreciation therefore needs to be subtracted from the net cash flow figures.

Staying with the example used for the pay back period, and assuming annual depreciation of £1,000:

Year	Income £	Costs £	Depreciation £	Net profit £
1	4,000	2,500	1,000	500
2	6,000	3,000	1,000	2,000
3	6,000	3,000	1,000	2,000
4	6,000	3,000	1,000	2,000
5	6,000	3,000	1,000	2,000
Total net profit over 5 years				**8,500**

Average annual net profit 1,700

$$\text{Annual rate of return} = \frac{£1,700}{£10,000} \times 100 = 17\%$$

When deciding between projects, the one offering the highest rate of return would be preferred. Any proposed investment should achieve a minimum rate of return of say 10% or 15%, as this level of return could be achieved more safely by investing in stocks and shares, or leaving the money on deposit at the bank.

Net Present Value

Two problems with the annual rate of return are:

❏ it takes no account of the timings of returns (i.e. whether the money is received next year or in five years)
❏ the fact that money today is worth more than money to be received in the future, because of:
   (a) inflation, that reduces the buying power of money over time, *and*
   (b) interest that could be received on money that is placed on deposit at a bank.

To allow for these effects of inflation and interest, discount factors are used to reduce the value of money to be received in the future. The appropriate discount factor to use can be found by reference to tables such as the one in Figure 15.1. This shows, for example, that £1 in three years' time, at a discount rate of 8%, will only be worth 79.4p.

Year	Discount rate (%)							
	6	8	10	12	14	16	18	20
1	0.943	0.926	0.909	0.893	0.877	0.862	0.847	0.833
2	0.890	0.857	0.826	0.797	0.769	0.743	0.718	0.694
3	0.840	**0.794**	0.751	0.712	0.675	0.641	0.609	0.579
4	0.792	0.735	0.683	0.636	0.592	0.552	0.516	0.482
5	0.747	0.681	0.621	0.567	0.519	0.476	0.437	0.402
6	0.705	0.630	0.564	0.507	0.456	0.410	0.370	0.335
7	0.665	0.583	0.513	0.452	0.400	0.354	0.314	0.279
8	0.627	0.540	0.467	0.404	0.351	0.305	0.266	0.233
9	0.592	0.500	0.424	0.361	0.308	0.263	0.225	0.194
10	0.558	0.463	0.386	0.322	0.270	0.227	0.191	0.162

Figure 15.1   Table of discount factors – future value of £1

The net present value of a project is worked out by:

NPV = value of the future net cash flows (discounted) minus initial investment

To continue with the example, the net present value calculation, using discount factors at 8%, would be:

Year	Investment £	Net cash flow £	Discount factor 8%	Net present value £
0	(10,000)		1.000	(10,000)
1		1,500	0.926	1,389
2		3,000	0.857	2,572
3		3,000	0.794	2,381
4		3,000	0.735	2,205
5		3,000	0.681	2,042
Net present value				589

The appropriate rate of discount factor to use is based on likely rates of inflation and interest. If the net present value is positive at this discount rate, then the investment would be financially worthwhile. When the choice is between two or more projects, the one giving the highest net present value would be chosen.

Internal Rate of Return

The internal rate of return is defined as 'the discount rate, which, when applied to a project's future cash flows, yields a net present value of zero'. Or, more simply, it is the rate of return after allowing for the fact that money in the future is worth less than today.

Finding the internal rate of return (IRR) is a matter of trial and error. The simplest method is to calculate the net present value at two different discount rates, with hopefully one giving a positive and the other a negative result. The answer can then be found by means of a graph.

If a discount rate of 12% is applied to the example, the result is as follows:

Year	Investment £	Net cash flow £	Discount factor 12%	Net present value £
0	(10,000)		1.000	(10,000)
1		1,500	0.893	1,339
2		3,000	0.797	2,392
3		3,000	0.712	2,135
4		3,000	0.636	1,907
5		3,000	0.567	1,702
Net present value				**(525)**

The graph to find the IRR is shown in Figure 15.2.

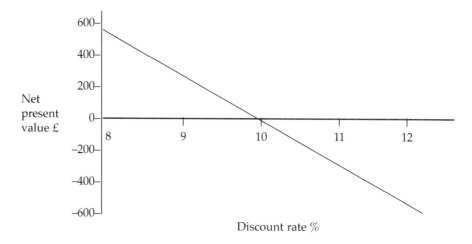

Figure 15.2   Graph to find the internal rate of return

From the graph it can be deduced that the NPV is 0 at a discount rate of just over 10%, giving an IRR of say 10.1%.

The higher the IRR, the more satisfactory the investment. A business is likely to set a minimum rate which a project should achieve before it is considered worthwhile, as with the annual rate of return.

Case Study

Linda has now been running her business for two years, and is pleased with progress to date. She is considering expanding by investing in six more stables for full liveries. Details of the proposal are:

	£
Investment – buildings	15,000
Expected net cash flows	
Year 1	2,000
2	6,000
3	6,000
4	6,000
5	6,000

Applying the investment appraisal techniques shows the following:

(1) Pay back period

	£
Investment	15,000
Cumulative net cash flow	
Year 1	2,000
2	8,000
3	14,000
4	20,000
Pay back period (years)	3.2

The project achieves a pay back in just over three years.

(2)   Annual rate of return

Assuming depreciation on the buildings is £1,500 per year, the annual net profits will be:

Year	Net cash flow £	Net profit £
1	2,000	500
2	6,000	4,500
3	6,000	4,500
4	6,000	4,500
5	6,000	4,500
		18,500
Average annual net profit		**3,700**

The annual rate of return can now be calculated:

$$\text{Annual rate of return} = \frac{£3,700}{£15,000} \times 100$$

$$= 24.7\%$$

Hence the proposal shows a high rate of return.

(3) Net present value

Linda considers that a discount rate of 10% is appropriate, given current interest and inflation rates. The calculations are:

Year	Net cash flow £	Discount factor	NPV £
0	(15,000)	1.000	(15,000)
1	2,000	0.909	1,818
2	6,000	0.826	4,959
3	6,000	0.751	4,508
4	6,000	0.683	4,098
5	6,000	0.621	3,726
Net present value			**4,109**

This NPV figure is positive, suggesting that the proposal is worth pursuing.

(4) Internal rate of return

To arrive at the IRR, Linda first of all calculated the NPV using a discount rate of 20%, and obtained a result of –£390. She then prepared the graph in Figure 15.3.

From the graph the IRR can be estimated as 19.1%, which is an acceptable return.

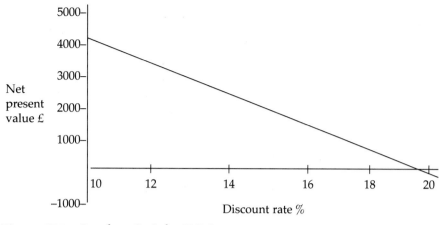

Figure 15.3   Graph to find the IRR for investment in stables

Exercise

As an alternative to using the extra stables for full liveries, Linda is also considering the possibility of increasing the number of school horses. Details of this option are:

		£
Investment – Buildings		15,000
Horses		9,000
Tack		3,000
		27,000

Expected net cash flows

Year	1	5,000
	2	11,000
	3	11,000
	4	11,000
	5	11,000

(1) Apply the following investment appraisal techniques to this option:
(a) Pay back period
(b) Annual rate of return – depreciation £1,500 per year
(c) Net present value, using a discount factor of 10%
(d) Internal rate of return – calculate the NPV using a discount rate of 20% to assist with this.

(2) Suggest, with reasons, which of the two options Linda should choose to invest in.

Part 3

Looking Back – What Happened?

Analysis of Business Performance

Chapter 16
How are we Doing?
An Initial View of Performance

It is important to look back at the performance of a business, to see how it is getting on.

❑ Are the objectives being met, such as the repayment of borrowing, or an adequate return to the owner?
❑ If it continues on the present course, what is likely to happen in the future?

The accounts and other records need to be examined to see what lessons can be learnt. Various techniques are available, including SWOT analysis and comparative analysis.

SWOT Analysis

SWOT stands for:

Strengths	what the business is doing well and should try to build on
Weaknesses	aspects of the business that are not up to standard, and which need to be improved or eliminated
Opportunities	factors in the business environment that provide the business with a chance to develop
Threats	external influences that are likely to make life more difficult, such as recession, or changes in the law.

Hence strengths and weaknesses are concerned with what is happening within the business and are under the control of the manager. Opportunities and threats are changes in the wider economy that the manager needs to be aware of and react to in an appropriate way.

Comparative Analysis

The latest year's results can be compared in several ways:

❑ against the budget for the year
❑ with the results of previous years
❑ with results from similar businesses, or management 'standards'.

Key Aspects of Performance

At its simplest level, looking at business performance will focus on three key areas of the business finances. These are:

- ❏ profitability
- ❏ cash flow
- ❏ capital value.

Profit

It is vital that a business makes a profit. If it does not make an adequate amount then it will fail, unless the owner can afford to keep injecting personal money to maintain it. A key word here is 'sufficient'. It is not satisfactory just to make some profit: there must be enough to meet all of the demands made upon it. The major factors to consider are:

- ❏ repayment of borrowing;
- ❏ reinvestment in the business, in the form of new buildings, facilities or vehicles;
- ❏ a return to the owner(s) of the business in the form of private drawings for a sole trader or partnership, or dividends to shareholders in a limited company;
- ❏ payment of any tax due on the profits made.

These four items are known as 'after profit expenses', because the business has to find sufficient money for them all out of the profits that it makes.

Cash flow

The cash flow of a business can be readily seen by looking at the change in bank balance over a period of time. It does not necessarily follow that the bank balance will improve if the business makes a profit – it can quite easily decline. There are many reasons for this, and they are explored in detail in the next chapter. The 'after profit expenses' mentioned above are major factors though.

Many profitable businesses fail, often because they run out of cash. It is vital to keep a careful eye on the bank balance, to make sure that the business always has enough ready money.

Capital

Perhaps the most reliable sign of when the business is doing well is that the net capital is increasing from one year to the next. This can be seen by looking at a series of balance sheets. If the value is declining this shows that the business is going downhill. If the trend cannot be reversed, then sooner or later the business will have to stop trading. Even if the net capital is increasing, there could still be cash flow problems.

Drawing Conclusions

It is very important, when looking at the performance of a business, not to jump to conclusions. All of the information needs to be assessed first. If the business is making a healthy profit, the bank balance is improving and the net capital increasing, then there is little to worry about. There are still likely to be areas for improvement, however.

If only one or two of the key areas of finance look satisfactory, then further investigation is needed. The business could be basically sound, but need to make a few small changes. Or it could be in a serious state of ill-health and need drastic action if it is going to survive.

Whatever the figures, two important questions to ask are:

❑ Has the business made *enough* profit?
❑ What are the reasons for the difference between net profit and net cash flow?

The techniques to find out the answers are described in the following chapters.

Case Study

Linda's accounts for her first two years of trading are shown in Figures 16.1 and 16.2.

The most important figures from these accounts, along with the budget figures, are summarised below.

Profitability

The first year shows a small loss, which was not unexpected. 1995/96 was much better, with a healthy net profit of over £25,000. The budget targets and actual results were:

Net profit	1995/6	1994/5
	£	£
Budget	22,918	(3,493)
Actual	25,261	(5,205)

The business was therefore close to the target in both years.

<u>Miss L. Clark, Oxhill Stables</u>
Balance sheets

	31 Mar 96	1 Apr 95	1 Apr 94
	£	£	£
Fixed assets			
Buildings	18,400	19,200	
Vehicles	4,500	6,000	8,000
Horses and ponies	18,900	21,500	
Tack and equipment	4,500	4,500	
	46,300	51,200	8,000
Current assets			
Feed stocks	220	190	
Debtors	350	170	
Bank balance			20,000
	570	360	20,000
Current liabilities			
Creditors	155	120	
Bank overdraft	1,849	19,495	
	2,004	19,615	0
Net current assets	**(1,434)**	**(19,255)**	**20,000**
Long-term liabilities			
Bank loan	12,000	16,000	0
Net capital	**32,866**	**15,945**	**28,000**
Financed by:			
Opening net capital	15,945	28,000	
+ Net profit	25,261	(5,205)	
– Private and tax	(8,340)	(6,850)	
Closing net capital	**32,866**	**15,945**	

Schedule of fixed assets 1994/5

	Initial cost	Value on 1/4/94	Deprec- iation	Deprec- iation	Value on 31/3/95
	£	£	%	£	£
Buildings	20,000	–	4	800	19,200
Vehicles		8,000	25	2,000	6,000

Schedule of fixed assets 1995/6

	Initial cost	Value on 1/4/95	Deprec- iation	Deprec- iation	Value on 31/3/96
	£	£	%	£	£
Buildings	20,000	19,200	4	800	18,400
Vehicles		6,000	25	1,500	4,500

Figure 16.1   Oxhill Stables balance sheets

Miss L. Clark, Oxhill Stables
Trading and profit and loss accounts for the years ending 31 March

	1996		1995	
	£	£	£	£
Sales				
Riding lessons	85,276		51,761	
Livery fees	19,762		16,238	
Sundry livery income	2,450		1,725	
		107,488		69,724
Less cost of sales				
Opening stock	21,690		0	
Horses and ponies	0		24,480	
Concentrate feed	9,403		7,837	
Hay	6,486		5,406	
Straw	3,347		2,574	
Farrier	2,380		2,094	
Veterinary and medicines	1,390		1,728	
Grassland expenses	275		257	
	44,971		44,376	
Less closing stock	(19,120)		(21,690)	
		25,851		22,686
Gross profit		**81,637**		**47,038**
Overheads				
Wages and NI		27,980		22,875
Rent		8,000		8,000
Rates		3,060		2,850
Water		560		524
Electricity		438		379
Vehicle expenses		2,680		2,185
Vehicle depreciation		1,500		2,000
Property repairs and maintenance		1,230		2,418
Buildings depreciation		800		800
Tack repairs and replacement		1,322		269
Insurance		2,310		1,563
Advertising		724		956
Telephone, office expenses and fees		1,774		2,314
Loan interest		2,240		2,800
Bank interest and charges		1,758		2,310
		56,376		52,243
Net profit		**25,261**		**(5,205)**

Figure 16.2   Oxhill Stables trading and profit and loss accounts

Cash flow

	1995/6 £	1994/5 £
Actual figures		
Closing bank balance	(1,849)	(19,495)
Opening bank balance	(19,495)	20,000
Net cash flow	17,646	(39,495)
Budgeted figures		
Closing bank balance	(5,309)	(20,560)
Opening bank balance	(20,560)	20,000
Net cash flow	15,251	(40,560)

Net cash flow = closing bank balance minus opening bank balance.

A large cash deficit in the first year was anticipated, with high initial costs and time taken for trade to build up. The second year showed a large reduction in the overdraft, to under £2,000. This was over £3,000 better than the budget.

Capital

The actual and budgeted net capital figures are:

	31/3/96 £	1/4/96 £	1/4/94 £
Actual	32,866	15,945	28,000
Budget	30,424	16,507	28,000

Again, the second year shows a healthy increase in the value of the business, better than the budget.

Conclusions

The first year was difficult, with a lot of expenses to get the business started, and time taken for trade to build up. Year two was much better, with the budget targets beaten, a healthy profit, and the overdraft nearly paid off. If it can continue at the current level, the business will be able to repay its debts and provide a reasonable living for Linda.

This discussion can be taken a step further, to try and answer some unresolved questions from the analysis. Using the figures for 1994/5:

❑   Why did the value of the business decline from £28,000 to £15,945 – a fall of £12,055, when the business only made a loss of £5,205?

❑   Why did the bank balance go down by £40,560, when the loss for the year was £5,205?

The answer to the first question is given in the capital account, or 'Financed by' section of the balance sheet. This shows that the fall in capital value is due to:

❑ the loss of £5,205, *and*
❑ the private drawings taken out the business.

To explain the difference between the net cash flow and net profit for the year is more difficult, but can be done using the technique of 'sources and applications of funds'. This is the subject of the next chapter. Obvious factors that will have contributed to the situation are:

❑ private drawings of   £6,850
❑ investment in buildings   £20,000
❑ purchase of horses and ponies   £24,480

The situation, and initial explanation, is summarised in Figure 16.3.

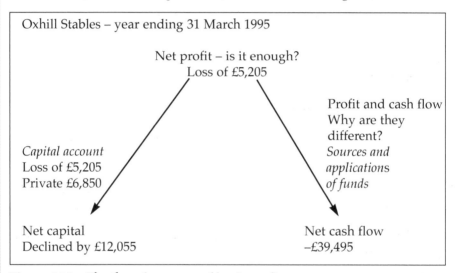

Figure 16.3 inner content:

Oxhill Stables – year ending 31 March 1995

Net profit – is it enough?
Loss of £5,205

Profit and cash flow
Why are they
different?
*Sources and
applications
of funds*

Capital account
Loss of £5,205
Private £6,850

Net capital
Declined by £12,055

Net cash flow
–£39,495

Figure 16.3   The three key areas of business finance

Chapter 17
Money in and Money out
The Cash Flow Statement

'The accountant says I made £20,000, but the overdraft has gone up by £10,000 – I don't understand it.' This is a predicament that often occurs, and there are a number of reasons why it can happen. These will determine whether there is cause for concern or not.

A key point is that profit is not the same as money in the bank. Major factors in this are the 'after profit expenses' referred to in the previous chapter, but other influences can include:

❏ an increase in the value of stocks
❏ changes in debtors or creditors
❏ depreciation.

The aim of a cash flow statement is to show why the profit and cash flow are different. It illustrates how the business has used its cash over the year, something that the balance sheet and trading and profit and loss (TP&L) account fail to do. This information can be very useful when assessing the performance of the business, especially showing whether it is managing to generate enough money.

Sources and Applications of Funds

The simplest form of cash flow statement is prepared by listing sources and applications of funds.

❏ Sources – ways in which money has come into the business, or cash generators.
❏ Applications – where the money has gone to, or cash users.

The difference between these will equal the change in the business bank balance over the year, i.e:

Sources of funds minus applications of funds = net cash flow
(i.e. closing bank balance minus opening bank balance)

Items that are included under each heading are shown in Figure 17.1. Not all of these will be relevant in every situation, but by carefully going through the balance sheets and TP&L account the appropriate figures can be extracted.

Sources of funds (Cash generators)	Applications of funds (Cash users)
Net profit	Net loss
Decrease in stocks value	Increase in stocks value
Decrease in debtors	Increase in debtors
Increase in creditors	Decrease in creditors
Capital sales and grants	Capital payments (investments)
Depreciation	
Loans taken out	Loan repayments
Funds introduced – private money or share issues	Private drawings/dividends
	Tax payments

Figure 17.1   Sources and applications of funds

Why do different items appear under the headings of sources or applications?

❑ Profit puts value into the business, while a loss has the opposite effect.
❑ An increase in stock value means that the business has tied up its money in physical assets, so reducing its supply of cash. A decrease in stock will release cash.
❑ Debtors increasing means that the business is owed more money by customers. These sales are included in the TP&L account, but the money is still with the customer rather than being in the business bank account. A decrease in debtors returns cash to the business.
❑ Changes in creditors have the opposite effect. An increase in creditors means that the money is still with the business, rather than having been paid to the suppliers. While this improves the bank position, it is not sound business practice.
❑ Capital sales and payments involve an inflow or outflow of cash.
❑ Depreciation – although it is included as an expense in the TP&L account, the money has not actually been spent. It is therefore still available to the business to spend in some other way.
❑ Loans taken out have the effect of putting money into the business bank account, although it will usually be quickly spent on something.

After preparing the sources and applications of funds statement, it is possible to identify the reasons for the change in bank balance. When looking at a poor cash flow, factors to consider are:

❑ Is it due to insufficient profit? This should be at least as much as the private drawings, tax and any loan repayments added together.
❑ Have capital investments taken place? This could make the cash flow

look unhealthy for one year, or it may be that too much money is being spent.
❑ Customers that have not paid may be starving the business of cash.

Larkhill Stables – sources and applications of funds statement for the year ending 30 September 199_

Sources of funds	£	Applications of funds	£
Net profit	12,000	Loan repayment	7,000
Increase in creditors	2,000	Capital investment	5,000
Depreciation	4,000	Private drawings	10,000
		Income tax	1,500
	18,000		23,500
Net cash flow	(5,500)		

Figure 17.2   A sources and applications of funds statement for Larkhill Stables

Figure 17.2 shows an example sources and applications of funds statement. The main points to note from this are:

❑ The bank balance has declined by £5,500.
❑ This is because the profit is insufficient to meet the loan repayment, private drawings and tax, which together total £18,500.
❑ The business therefore has problems and needs to increase its profitability to about £20,000 if it is to be secure.
❑ The position would have been worse had creditors not increased, but this is an unhealthy way to control the bank balance.

Modern Cash Flow Statements

Since 1991, a standard layout for cash flow statements has been used. This focuses on cash movements, and places different cash flows under five headings. The layout is illustrated in Figure 17.3.

Larkhill Stables – cash flow statement for the year ending 30 Sept 199_

	£	£
Operating activities		
Net profit (before tax and interest)	13,000	
+ depreciation	4,000	
+ decrease (–increase) in stocks	...	
+ decrease (–increase) in debtors	...	
+ increase (–decrease) in creditors	2,000	
Net cash inflow (outflow) from operating activities		19,000
Returns on investments and servicing of finance		
+ interest received	...	
– interest paid	(1,000)	
+ dividends received	...	
– dividends paid/private drawings	(10,000)	
Net cash inflow (outflow) from returns on investments and servicing of finance		(11,000)
Taxation		
– tax paid		(1,500)
Investing activities		
+ receipts from sales of fixed assets	...	
– payments to acquire fixed assets	(5,000)	
Net cash inflow (outflow) from investing activities		(5,000)
Financing		
+ issue of share capital	...	
– repayment of capital	...	
+ increase (–repayment) of loans	(7,000)	
Net cash inflow (outflow) from financing		(7,000)
Increase (decrease) in cash		(5,500)
Analysis of changes in cash during the year		
Balance of cash and bank at start of year		3,200
+ net cash inflow (outflow)		(5,500)
Balance of cash and bank at end of year		(2,300)

Figure 17.3   Layout of a cash flow statement

Case Study

The sources and applications of funds statement for Oxhill Stables, for the year ending 31 March 1995, is shown below.

Sources of funds		Applications of funds	
	£		£
Depreciation	2,800	Loss	5,205
Loan taken out	20,000	Increase in stocks	21,690
Increase in creditors	120	Increase in debtors	170
		Loan repayment	4,000
		Private and tax	6,850
		Capital investments	24,500
	22,920		62,415

Decrease in bank balance (39,495)

Closing bank balance	(19,495)
Opening bank balance	20,000
	(39,495)

This shows that the bank balance decreased by nearly £40,000. The main reasons are that the business made a loss, at the same time as investing a considerable sum of money in stock and buildings. This was necessary to get the enterprise started, and so a decrease in bank balance was inevitable.

Exercises

(1) Details for two businesses, for the year ending 31 March 199_, are shown below.

	Business	
	A	B
	£	£
Net profit	18,000	6,000
Private drawings	11,000	7,000
Tax	3,000	0
Capital investment	12,000	2,500
Depreciation	5,000	3,000
Increase in debtors	2,000	20
Increase (decrease) in stocks	3,000	(4,000)
Increase in creditors	0	2,000

(a) Prepare the sources and applications of funds statements for each business.

(b) Comment on the performance of each.

(2) Referring to the accounts for Linda Clark shown in the previous chapter, prepare the sources and applications of funds statement for the year ending 31 March 1996. The items to include are the same as in the case study except:

❑   there will be no 'Loan taken out' or 'Capital investments'
❑   the business made a net profit rather than a loss.

Chapter 18
A Capital Position?
Detailed Study of the Balance Sheet

The balance sheet shows how much a business is worth. It can also indicate how secure it is, especially when statements covering several years are available. These need to reflect the current value of the business, rather than dated values which can often be found on the accountant's report. To provide the figures it is helpful to prepare a balance sheet for management purposes, based on market values, at the end of each financial year.

Analysis of the balance sheet will consist of two activities:

❏ a study of the absolute figures and trends over time
❏ the calculation of ratios from the figures.

Trends in Assets and Liabilities

The most important trend was noted in chapter 16 – what is happening to the net capital of the business? In a healthy situation it will be increasing, and if this is not the case then there are problems that need to be addressed. Other points to look for:

❏ There is an adequate level of working capital (net current assets).
❏ The bank balance is under control, and preferably increasing over time.
❏ The fixed assets of the business are being maintained by regular, sensible, investment.
❏ Loans are being repaid on time.
❏ There is a sensible balance between fixed and current assets. This will depend very much on the nature of the business, but the aim should be to have money in income generating assets rather than an excessive amount of long-term fixtures.

A study of these points will show if the business is being maintained and in a healthy condition.

Balance Sheet Ratios

A problem with the figures on the balance sheet is that they are difficult to relate to the size of the business. For example, a net capital of £250,000 would be high for a small business, but very low for a large one. Ratios seek to overcome this problem.

Different calculations can be made to assess the strength of the business in the long term and the short term. The balance sheet in Figure 18.1, which was referred to in chapter 4, will be used to illustrate the different ratios.

Windmill Stables – balance sheet on 31 March 199_

	£	£
Fixed assets		
Buildings and fixtures	15,360	
Machinery and vehicles	11,400	
Brood mares	3,000	
		29,760
Current assets		
Young horses	10,800	
Stores of feed	250	
Debtors	2,240	
Bank balance	200	
	13,490	
Current liabilities		
Creditors	1,420	
Bank overdraft	3,202	
	4,622	
Net current assets		**8,868**
Long-term liability		
Bank loan		3,000
Net capital		**35,628**
Financed by:		
Opening net capital		34,380
Add: Net profit for the year		13,028
		47,208
Subtract: Private drawings		(11,780)
		35,628

Figure 18.1   Balance sheet for Windmill Stables

Long-term Strength (Solvency)

This is concerned with the ability of the business to continue into the future, and survive difficult times if the need arises.

Owner Equity Percentage

The owner equity percentage looks at the proportion of the assets of the business that are funded by the owner's capital, rather than borrowing. It is found by the formula:

$$\text{Owner equity } \% = \frac{\text{net capital}}{\text{total assets}} \times 100$$

A high figure suggests that the business is secure and able to withstand hard times. It should also have little trouble if it wants to borrow for sensible investments. If the figure is low, the business is vulnerable to collapse if it experiences a period of low profits. Because of its dependence on borrowed money, it will also suffer from high interest rates. Lenders would be unwilling to finance such a business.

For Windmill Stables, the calculation is:

$$\text{Owner equity } \% = \frac{£35,628}{£43,250 \text{ (i.e. } £29,760 + £13,490)} \times 100 = 82\%$$

As the value of the premises is not included in the assets, this would be considered a high figure.

General guidelines for a minimum acceptable level of owner equity percent are:

- over 80% if property value is included
- 67% if it is not.

Capital gearing

Another long term measure is the capital gearing ratio. This only includes the long term liabilities, which represent a commitment to repay capital and interest over a number of years. It is calculated by the formula:

Capital gearing = loans : net capital

It can also be expressed as a percentage:

$$\text{Capital gearing} = \frac{\text{loan capital}}{\text{net capital}} \times 100$$

If the ratio is greater than 1:1, or 100%, the business is considered to be highly geared. This represents a situation with significant risk, as a large proportion of the income will go on financing the borrowing. In hard times, a highly geared business is more likely to fail.

The gearing ratio for Windmill Stables is:

Capital gearing = £3,000 : £35,628 = 1:12

or $\dfrac{£3,000 \times 100}{£35,628} = 8\%$

This business has a low gearing.

Short-term Strength (Liquidity)

Liquidity is how well placed the business is to pay its way in the short-term. Running out of available money can be a major problem and result in the failure of an otherwise sound business. Again, two different ratios are calculated.

Current ratio

The current ratio, or working capital ratio as it is sometimes known, looks at the ability of the business to pay its debts from production that is in process. The result is expressed as a percentage using the formula:

$$\text{Current ratio} = \frac{\text{current assets}}{\text{current liabilities}} \times 100$$

A generally recommended figure is 200%, indicating that there are £2 worth of assets for each £1 of liabilities. This means that it is often unwise to operate a business on a large overdraft: a smaller overdraft and the remainder of the borrowing on a fixed term loan would be better.

For Windmill Stables, the current ratio is:

$$\text{Current ratio} = \frac{£13,490}{£4,622} \times 100 = 292\%$$

This is comfortably above the recommended level of 200%.

Liquidity ratio

The second short-term measure is the liquidity ratio, also known as the quick, or acid test ratio. This examines the immediate ability of the business to meet its current liabilities, by looking at the level of liquid assets. These are the assets which are already cash, or very quickly will be, and include:

❏   cash on hand or at the bank
❏   outstanding debtors (assuming that they will pay soon).

$$\text{Liquidity ratio} = \frac{\text{liquid assets}}{\text{current liabilities}} \times 100$$

The usual guideline is that this figure should be more than 100%, showing that the business can pay back its short-term borrowing at short notice.

The figure for Windmill Stables is:

$$\text{Liquidity ratio} = \frac{£2,420}{£4,622} \times 100 = 52\%$$

This is well below the guideline minimum.

Many businesses manage to operate successfully with a low liquidity ratio. It is only likely to be serious if there is a real prospect of the current liabilities having to be repaid at short notice, and this situation usually builds up over a period of time:

❏ The business struggles to generate enough money
❏ The bank balance gradually falls
❏ After a point the bank manager puts a limit on the overdraft
❏ Debts to creditors then start to rise
❏ Sooner or later the crunch comes – drastic action has to be taken to acquire some money or the business must fold.

This type of situation is known as a liquidity crisis, and its development needs to be spotted early.

It is not only the struggling business that needs to keep a careful eye on its liquidity position. Another scenario where a liquidity crisis can occur is in a rapidly expanding business, when all of the available cash has been tied up in stock and investments. This is known as overtrading, and usually occurs when a business tries to grow too quickly.

Return on Capital

A final ratio to calculate from the balance sheet links it with the TP&L account. This is the return on capital employed, which looks at the return, in the form of net profit, that is being generated from the money invested in the business. It is calculated by the formula:

$$\text{Return on capital employed} = \frac{\text{net profit}}{\text{capital employed}} \times 100$$

The capital employed is the money tied up in the business long-term, and is the net capital plus the long-term liabilities.

Capital employed = net capital plus long-term liabilities

The result can be compared with alternative uses for the money, to see if it is making a worthwhile return.

The return for Windmill Stables is:

$$\text{Return on capital employed} = \frac{£13,028}{£38,628} \times 100 = 34\%$$

This is a very high level of return which would be difficult to better in any other form of investment.

Use of Ratios

Ratios need to be used carefully, bearing in mind that:

❑ a figure must never be viewed in isolation, but in the context of all the other information about the business;
❑ trends can be as significant, if not more so, than the ratios themselves;
❑ it is the story behind the figures that is most important.

However, they are a useful way of spotting problems in a business, and indicating areas of strength.

Case Study

Analysis of Linda's balance sheets, shown in chapter 16, reveals the following:

	31/3/96	31/3/95
Owner equity %	£32,866	£15,945
	£46,870	£51,560
	= 70%	= 31%
Capital gearing	£12,000	£16,000
	£32,866	£15,945
	= 36%	= 100%

These show a high level of borrowing, but one which is declining. The business needs to continue to make healthy profits if it is to become more secure.

	31/3/96	31/3/95
Current ratio	£570	£360
	£2,004	£19,615
	= 28%	= 2%
Liquidity ratio	£350	£170
	£2,004	£19,615
	= 17%	= 1%

Both of these ratios are low but improving. There should be no problem in keeping the support of the bank manager if the business continues to perform as it has for the year ending 31 March 1996.

	31/3/96	**31/3/95**
Return on capital employed	£25,261	(£5,205)
	£44,866	£31,945
	= 56%	= (7%)

The figure for the later year is very high. If this level of profit can be sustained in the future, the other ratios will quickly improve.

Exercise

The balance sheets for Larkhill Stables are shown in Figure 18.1. From these balance sheets:

(1) Comment on the trends between the two sets of figures.

(2) Calculate the following ratios:
  Owner equity %
  Capital gearing ratio
  Current ratio
  Liquidity ratio
  Return on capital employed (for the year ending 30 September 1996).
  Comment on the significance of these calculations.

Balance sheets for Larkhill Stables

	30 Sept 1996		1 Oct 1995	
	£	£	£	£
Fixed assets				
Premises	200,000		200,000	
Vehicles	13,500		12,000	
		213,500		212,000
Current assets				
Horses	11,000		10,000	
Stocks of materials	300		450	
Debtors	375		745	
	11,675		11,195	
Current liabilities				
Bank overdraft	11,510		6,000	
Creditors	690		745	
	12,200		6,745	
Net current assets		(525)		4,450
Long-term liability				
Mortgage		40,000		40,000
Net capital		172,975		176,450
Financed by:				
Net capital on 1/10/95		176,450		
Net profit		9,400		
Private drawings and tax		(12,875)		
Net capital on 30/9/96		172,975		

Figure 18.1 Larkhill Stables balance sheets

Chapter 19
Effort and Efficiency
Further Measures of Business Performance

A number of other calculations can also be made on the accounts. These all try to indicate areas of strength or weakness in different aspects of the business's finances. They can be used to compare the performance of the business against previous years, or to other similar businesses. Data on a range of horse enterprises, to enable this comparison, is available in the *Equine Business Guide*.

Profitability

In addition to the return on capital employed, the gross profit and net profit percentages can be calculated.

Gross profit percentage

This is derived by the formula:

$$\text{Gross profit percentage} = \frac{\text{gross profit}}{\text{sales revenue}} \times 100$$

For example, referring to the trading and profit and loss account for Windmill Stables, which was introduced in chapter 4 and is shown in Figure 19.1.

$$\text{Gross profit percentage} = \frac{£50,346}{£68,650} \times 100 = 73\%$$

Hence each £1 of sales is producing 73p of gross profit.

This calculation needs to be carried out regularly. A fall shows that costs may have increased or prices fallen. Action should be taken to try and raise prices or control costs.

Windmill Stables – trading and profit and loss account for the year ending 31 March 199_

	£	£
Sales		
Livery fees	52,710	
Sales of youngsters	12,400	
Sundry livery income	3,540	
		68,650
Less cost of sales		
Opening stock	12,400	
Feed	7,554	
Bedding	3,684	
Hay	6,286	
Veterinary and medicines	890	
Farriery	120	
Stud fees and mare's livery	1,020	
Contractors – grassland maintenance	400	
	32,354	
Less closing stock	(14,050)	
		18,304
Gross profit		**50,346**
Overheads		
Paid labour	15,288	
Rent	7,000	
Rates and water	2,800	
Machinery and vehicles expenses	6,160	
Property repairs and maintenance	1,620	
Insurance	980	
Accountancy	800	
Office and administration expenses	1,700	
Bank interest and charges	970	
		37,318
Net profit for the year		**13,028**

Figure 19.1   Trading and profit and loss account for Windmill Stables

Net profit percentage

The formula to calculate net profit percentage is very similar:

$$\text{Net profit percentage} = \frac{\text{net profit}}{\text{sales revenue}} \times 100$$

It may fall because of a lower gross profit percentage, or if the overhead expenses increase. Thus it can show if more careful cost control is needed.

The figure for Windmill Stables is:

$$\text{Net profit percentage} = \frac{£13,028}{£68,650} \times 100 = 19\%$$

This is a reasonably high result.

Debtors and Creditors

The time taken to receive money from customers and make payment to suppliers can have a significant impact on the cash position of a business. Customers who pay late can cause serious liquidity problems.

Credit given

The period of credit given is calculated in the following way:

$$\text{Average credit given} = \frac{\text{debtors} \times 365}{\text{sales}} \text{ days}$$

Example
Sales for the year are £100,000, and the average level of debtors £8,000.

$$\text{Average credit given} = \frac{£8,000 \times 365}{£100,000} = 29 \text{ days}$$

This figure can be related to the credit terms offered to customers, to see if they are being abused. Aged debtor lists should also be regularly checked to spot individual poor payers. It is desirable to be paid as quickly as possible.

Credit taken

The other side of the coin is the days of credit taken from suppliers. Here the business will wish to take the maximum benefit from any credit period offered. The formula is:

$$\text{Average credit taken} = \frac{\text{creditors} \times 365}{\text{purchases}} \text{ days}$$

Example
Purchases are £65,000, and the average level of creditors £6,000

$$\text{Average credit taken} = \frac{£6,000 \times 365}{£65,000} = 34 \text{ days}$$

Stock Turnover

It is unwise for a business to have too much money tied up in stock. This measure looks at the time taken for stock to be either used or sold.

$$\text{Stock turnover} = \frac{\text{cost of sales}}{\text{average stock}}$$

Example
Average stock (from the opening and closing balance sheets) is £10,000, and the cost of sales £120,000.

$$\text{Stock turnover} = \frac{£120,000}{£10,000} = 12 \text{ times}$$

The whole stock is being used (or sold) 12 times during the year, or once a month. To convert the result to days, divide 365 by the answer, which in the example gives a figure of:

$$\frac{365 \text{ days}}{12} = 30 \text{ days}$$

This figure will be important for enterprises such as a dealing yard or tack shop, where stock for sale represents a large sum of money. Any reduction in the stock turnover is likely to be serious for the business.

Finance Charges

Finance charges can significantly affect the level of profit achieved. This is measured by interest cover, which relates interest charges to profitability.

$$\text{Interest cover} = \frac{\text{profit before interest}}{\text{interest charges}} \times 100$$

Example
Interest charges (on loans, overdrafts and any other form of borrowing) are £10,000, and net profit (after interest) £40,000.

$$\text{Interest cover} = \frac{£50,000^*}{£10,000} \times 100 = 500\%$$

*i.e. £40,000 net profit plus £10,000 interest

A suggested guideline as a minimum is 300%. If the figure is less than 100%, interest charges exceed the profit made by the business.

Case Study

Relevant figures to calculate from Linda's accounts are:

Year ending 31 March	1996	1995
Gross profit %	$\dfrac{81,637}{107,488}$	$\dfrac{47,038}{69,724}$
	= 76%	= 67%

This has increased due to extra sales, especially from the riding school.

Net profit %	$\dfrac{25,261}{107,488}$	$\dfrac{(5,205)}{69,724}$
	= 24%	= (7%)

24% represents a high level of profitability.

Interest cover	$\dfrac{29,259}{3,998}$	$\dfrac{(95)}{5,110}$
	= 732%	= (2)%

Interest charges were not fully covered in the first year, but are now at a level that the business can support.

Conclusions

The latest figures all indicate that the business is performing well, and has shown significant improvement in the second year.

Exercise

From the accounts data in Figure 19.2, calculate for both years:

(1) gross profit and net profit percentages
(2) stock turnover
(3) credit given and credit taken
(4) interest cover.

Comment on the performance of the business.

Trading and profit and loss accounts for Top Tack Shop

Year ending 30 September	£	1996 £	£	1995 £
Sales		124,000		117,150
Less cost of sales:				
Opening stock	6,500		5,800	
Stock purchases	75,640		69,120	
(Closing stock)	(8,000)		(6,500)	
		74,140		68,420
Gross profit		**49,860**		**48,730**
Overheads	34,080		30,700	
Interest	2,000		1,500	
		36,080		32,200
Net profit		**13,780**		**16,530**
Average trade creditors		3,200		3,500
Average debtors		1,300		900

Figure 19.2   Trading and profit and loss account for Top Tack Shop.

Chapter 20
Is Everything Pulling its Weight?
Enterprise Analysis

Many businesses are made up of more than one activity, or enterprise. So far, ways of analysing the performance of the business as a whole have been studied, but it may be that one enterprise is letting the remainder down. The component parts need to be examined, as well as the overall business.

Gross Margin Analysis

This looks at the gross margin generated by each part of the business. The starting point is to construct gross margin statements to show the performance of each enterprise. These will be very similar to the gross margin budgets described in chapter 8. Information for this will come from the accounts and other records. The major difference, compared to gross margin budgets, is that valuation changes are also included. The statement will be calculated for the whole enterprise, and the figures then divided to show the performance per horse.

Example
A stud with ten mares
Gross margin for the year ending 31 March 199_

	Total	Per mare
	£	£
Sales		
Sales of youngsters	13,500	1,350
Variable costs		
Feed	1,500	150
Bedding	800	80
Hay	1,200	120
Veterinary and farrier	1,800	180
Stud fees	2,800	280
Grassland expenses	200	20
(Increase) in stock value	(2,000)	(200)
	6,300	630
Enterprise gross margin	**7,200**	**720**

The statement is most useful if measures of physical performance are also included, not only financial data. These would be details such as number of lessons per horse for a riding school, or mares covered per stallion in a stud. For the above example:

Performance measures

Foaling rate	90%
Average sale price	£1,500

Having prepared the data, it can be compared in four different ways to identify strengths and weaknesses.

❏ To the budget targets, to see if they have been met.
❏ Against results from previous years to discover whether the business is progressing. Consider whether an improvement is due to inflation or efficiency – has the school horses gross margin increased because of higher prices, or extra lessons?
❏ Compare the gross margins achieved by the different enterprises against each other. This may help to identify the most profitable areas of the business, which might then be expanded. Any enterprises that are weak financially may be replaced by one that is more rewarding. However, the enterprise with the highest gross margin is not necessarily the one that will produce the most net profit, as no account has been taken of overhead expenses.
❏ With standard data from other similar enterprises. This information is available in the *Equine Business Guide*.

For the example above, the information would be presented as follows:

	Total £	Per mare £	Standard £
Sales			
Sales of youngsters	13,500	1,350	2,250
Variable costs			
Feed	1,500	150	185
Bedding	800	80	64
Hay	1,200	120	152
Veterinary and farrier	1,800	180	214
Stud fee	2,800	280	385
Grassland expenses	200	20	44
Other			88
Valuation (increase)/decrease	(2,000)	(200)	191
	6,300	630	1,323
Enterprise gross margin	**7,200**	**720**	**927**
Performance measures			
Foaling rate		90%	80%
Average sale price		£1,500	£3,000

This analysis shows that:

❐   the gross margin is below average
❐   this is because of low sales
❐   variable costs are below average, even after allowing for the effects of stock value increases.

The business needs to try and improve by breeding better quality stock, or selling youngstock at an older age and higher price.

Complete Costing

A problem with gross margins, when trying to identify which parts of the business are most profitable, is that they take no account of overhead expenses. Complete costing seeks to overcome this by calculating a net margin figure for each enterprise. After calculating gross margins, the overhead expenses of the business are all allocated or apportioned between the enterprises.

❐   Allocation is when a cost is clearly related to only one activity. For example, advertising costs for a stallion, or a riding instructor's wages.
❐   Apportionment is used when costs are shared between a number of enterprises, which is usually the case with most of the overhead expenses. The cost is divided between the enterprises in proportion to:
    ❐   the number of horses
    ❐   or sales
    ❐   or some other arbitrary criteria.

A complete costing example for a riding school/livery business is shown below.

Data for the year ending 31 October 199_

	Total £	School £	Livery £
Sales/horse		5,000	3,000
Variable costs/horse		700	600
Gross margin/horse		4,300	2,400
Number of horses	25	15	10
Enterprise gross margin	**88,500**	**64,500**	**24,000**
Overhead expenses			
Rent and rates	10,000	6,000	4,000
Labour	30,000	18,000	12,000
Other	25,000	15,000	10,000
	65,000	39,000	26,000
Net margin	**23,500**	**25,500**	**(2,000)**

The overhead expenses have been apportioned in proportion to the number of horses.

Note: Apportionment of the overheads:

Rent and rates total £10,000

To school horses
$$\frac{£10,000 \times 15}{25} = £6,000$$

i.e. $£10,000 \times \dfrac{\text{number of school horses}}{\text{total number of horses}}$

The school horses have a higher gross margin, suggesting that they are more profitable than the livery horses. This is more clearly seen from the net margins. But is it reasonable to say that the livery is losing money?

❐ If the liveries are discontinued, most of their £26,000 of overhead expenses will still have to be paid.
❐ The business would actually be £24,000 worse off without them!
❐ Have the overhead expenses been apportioned fairly? If it was in proportion to the sales of the enterprises, the liveries would show a net profit.

While trying to overcome the limitations of gross margin analysis, complete costing obviously has problems of its own. On the positive side, it would help us to conclude, in the situation above, that:

❐ the school should be developed to its full potential
❐ after this point the liveries are making a useful contribution to the business net profit.

In practice it is usually best to work out gross margins. These can then be assessed in the awareness that different levels of overhead expenses may be involved with the various enterprises. A figure of gross margin minus labour cost would be straightforward to calculate, and useful, as labour is usually the largest item of overhead expenses.

Complete costing is most useful in a large yard, where a lot of the overheads can be clearly allocated to separate enterprises.

Overhead Expenses

Each enterprise may be performing well, but the business still fails to make adequate profits. This will be because the overhead expenses are too high.

The general situation will be shown by comparing the gross profit % and net profit % being achieved by the business with standard data from other similar businesses. The situation for a livery yard is given below:

	Per horse	Standard
	£	£
Sales	3,100	2,800
Variable costs	1,000	850
Gross margin	**2,100**	**1,950**
Overhead expenses	1,900	1,660
Net profit	**200**	**290**
Gross profit %	68	70
Net profit %	6	10

Gross margin compares well, but the net profit % is low, indicating a problem with the overhead expenses. Each item of overheads can be compared with the figure for the standard to try and identify the main areas that need reducing.

Case Study

To work out the gross margins achieved by the different parts of Linda's business, some more information is needed than that shown on the accounts. This is provided below for the year ending 31 March 1996.

	School horses	Ponies	Livery
Number of horses	8	6	8
	£	£	£
Sales			
Riding lessons	50,968	34,308	
Livery fees			19,762
Sundry livery income			2,450
Variable costs			
Concentrate feed	5,226	937	3,241
Hay	3,588	667	2,231
Straw	1,685	445	1,218
Farrier	1,600	780	
Veterinary and medicines	880	510	
Grassland expenses*	100	75	100

*The total of £275 divided equally between the 22 horses equals £12.50 per horse

Valuations			
Opening stock	16,020	5,670	
Closing stock	14,100	5,020	

School work	**Horses**	**Ponies**
Weeks of work	48	47
Average hours per week	13	11
Charge per hour (ex. VAT)	£10.21	£11.06

Livery uptake	**Full**	**DIY**
Weeks uptake	48	45
Charge per week (ex. VAT)	£63.83	£15.32

Using this information, the gross margin statements can now be prepared. The standard figures given are for illustrative purposes. Actual data from other horse businesses can be found in the *Equine Business Guide*.

Gross margin analysis for the year ending 31 March 1996
Riding school horses

	Total £	Per horse £	Budget £	Standard £
Sales				
Lessons	50,968	6,371	6,577	5,200
Variable costs				
Concentrate feed	5,226	653	568	350
Hay	3,588	449	390	220
Straw	1,685	211	234	150
Farrier	1,600	200	240	210
Veterinary and medicines	880	110	120	110
Grassland expenses	100	13	15	45
Horse replacement cost (valuation decrease)	1,980	248	266	220
	15,059	1,884	1,833	1,305
Enterprise gross margin	**35,909**	**4,487**	**4,744**	**3,895**
Performance measures				
Teaching hours/week		13	14	10
Lesson charge £/hour		10.21	10.21	10.00

Conclusions

Compared to the budget:

❐ Sales are lower because of less use from the horses.
❐ Variable costs are higher, especially concentrate feed and hay.
❐ Gross margin is lower as a result of the above.

Compared to the standard:

❐ Sales are higher because the horses have worked more hours at a higher price.

❑ Feed and bedding costs are significantly higher, probably reflecting the horses being stabled for more time.
❑ Despite this, the gross margin is £600 above the standard.

Gross margin analysis for the year ending 31 March 1996
Riding school ponies

	Total £	Per pony £	Budget £	Standard £
Sales				
Lessons	34,308	5,718	5,090	5,200
Variable costs				
Concentrate feed	937	156	142	350
Hay	667	111	117	220
Straw	445	74	78	150
Farrier	780	130	160	210
Veterinary and medicines	510	85	90	110
Grassland expenses	75	13	15	45
Replacement cost	650	108	150	220
	4,064	677	752	1,305
Enterprise gross margin	**30,244**	**5,041**	**4,338**	**3,895**
Performance measures				
Teaching hours/week		11	10	10
Lesson charge £/hour		11.06	11.06	10.00

Conclusions

Compared to the budget:

❑ Sales are higher because of more use from the ponies.
❑ Variable costs are similar, apart from farriery and the replacement cost, which are both lower.
❑ Gross margin is £700 higher.

Compared to the standard:

❑ Sales are higher because of an extra hour per week of teaching, and a higher average lesson charge.
❑ Variable costs are much lower, because the ponies are kept cheaply outside.
❑ The ponies achieve a gross margin over £1,000 better than average.

Gross margin analysis for the year ending 31 March 1996
Livery horses

	Total £	Per horse £	Budget £	Standard £
Sales				
Livery fees	19,762	2,470	2,872	2,730
Sundry livery income	2,450	306	250	300
	22,212	2,776	3,122	3,030
Variable costs				
Concentrate feed	3,241	405	490	320
Hay	2,231	279	338	210
Straw	1,218	152	203	110
Grassland expenses	100	13	15	40
	6,790	849	1,046	680
Enterprise gross margin	**15,422**	**1,927**	**2,076**	**2,350**
Performance measures				
Facility uptake (weeks)		47	45	42
Average charge £/week		52.55	63.83	65.00
Full livery		63.83		
DIY livery		15.32		

Conclusions

Compared to the budget:

❐ Sales are lower because of a reduced average livery fee.
❐ Variable costs are lower.
❐ The gross margin is £150 below the budget.

Compared to the standard:

❐ The facility uptake is higher by five weeks, but sales are low due to the lower average livery fee received.
❐ Variable costs are higher.
❐ The gross margin is therefore significantly lower than the standard.

Overall Conclusions

The riding school is performing well, with gross margins exceeding both the budgeted and standard figures. The livery enterprise appears to be the major weakness, with the horses achieving a below average gross margin, which is less than half that achieved by the school horses. Efforts need to be made to increase livery income and reduce costs.

Exercise

The following data apply to the accounts year ending 31 March 199_.

Sales	£
Riding lessons (12 horses)	49,680
Livery fees (8 horses)	24,960
School horse sold	600

Variable costs	Total	School	Livery
	£	£	£
Feed	5,000	3,120	1,880
Hay	5,600	3,360	2,240
Bedding	1,280	720	480
Veterinary and medicine	600	600	
Farrier	720	720	
Grassland	300	180	120

School horses – Opening valuation	10,200
Closing valuation	10,800
School horse purchased	1,500

(1) From this data calculate enterprise gross margins (per horse), for the year, for *both* the riding school and the livery horses.

(2) If the 'standard' gross margin per riding school horse is £3,900, suggest reasons why the gross margin for this business is different.

(3) Explain why the enterprise with the lowest gross margin is not necessarily the one that is least profitable.

Chapter 21

The Tax Man Cometh!

Taxation and the Horse Business

The manager is not the only person interested in the performance of the business, the tax authorities will also want to know, so that they can collect any revenues due to them.

A number of different taxes might have an impact on the business at some time or other, and these are outlined below. Only general details are given as this is a particularly difficult area on which to give impersonal advice. The position changes annually with the Chancellor of the Exchequer's budget, so any information soon becomes dated. Also, the advice will depend very much on individual circumstances. It is best therefore to consult an accountant on any specific matter that might have taxation implications.

Income Tax

The business owner may be affected by income tax in two ways.

Taxation of profits

If the business is run as a sole trader or partnership, then an income tax assessment will be made on the profit, or each partner's share of it. The Inland Revenue will apply strict rules as to what income is taxable and what expenditure is tax deductible. Some common problem areas are given here.

Horses for private use

These are not allowable as a business expense. A major area of difficulty is when a horse is kept partly for business and partly for private or recreational use. Here the costs of acquiring and keeping the horse must be apportioned, or divided, between the business and private expenses. Similarly, if a horse is entirely for private use, none of the costs of keep can be included as business expenses. If staff or transport costs are incurred on such horses, these must also be excluded from the accounts. In other words, the costs of keeping private horses have to be funded out of profits made, rather than being carried by the rest of the business.

Private use of vehicles

Again the costs need to be split between the business and private use, often on the basis of mileage for the different purposes.

Telephone and fuel/electricity expenses

If the business and private uses are not separately invoiced, the total costs have to be split and only the business proportion included as a cost to the business.

Allowances for capital expenditure (i.e. depreciation) are included in the accounts as an expense of the business. Limits to writing down allowances (or depreciation rates), for different types of capital investment, are set by the Chancellor of the Exchequer.

A number of legitimate ways of reducing a tax liability are available, such as by contributing to a personal pension plan.

When the amount of income tax due has been assessed, it will be payable in two instalments over the coming months. From 1996/7, the tax is assessed on the profit made in the accounts year ending in the current tax year, i.e:

Accounts for the year ending	30 June 1996
Assessed in tax year	1996/7
Tax payable	31 Jan 1997 and 31 July 1997

All businesses have to undertake self assessment of the amount of tax payable from April 1997. Penalties will be applied to late returns and interest charged on late payments. Records supporting the figures included in the tax return must be kept for six years after the date by which the return must have been made.

PAYE deductions from employees

It is the responsibility of the employer to collect any income tax due from employees. Failure to do this leaves the employer liable for the uncollected tax. The system used is called Pay As You Earn (PAYE), and involves any tax due being calculated every time an employee is paid.

The starting point for the calculations is the employee's tax code. To obtain the correct code, the employer needs to inform the local tax office of the name and National Insurance number of the employee. The code is based on the allowances, reliefs and taxable benefits of the individual, and represents the amount that they can earn free of tax during the year. For example, a single person, with personal allowance and reliefs of £3,515, would have the code 351L.

To assist with the calculations, booklets of tax tables are provided, examples of which are shown in Figure 21.1.

Table A – Pay adjustment

Code	Total pay adjustment to date	Code	Total pay adjustment to date	Code	Total pay adjustment to date	Code	Total pay adjustment to date	Code	Total pay adjustment to date
	£		£		£		£		£
121	23.45	181	34.99	241	46.52	301	58.06	351	67.68
122	23.64	182	35.18	242	46.72	302	58.25	352	67.87
123	23.83	183	35.37	243	46.92	303	58.45	353	68.06
124	24.02	184	35.56	244	47.10	304	58.64	354	68.25

Table B
(Tax at 25%)

Tax due on taxable pay from £1 to £99

Total taxable pay to date	Total tax due to date	Total taxable pay to date	Total tax due to date
£	£	£	£
1	0.25	61	15.25
2	0.50	62	15.50
3	0.75	63	15.75
4	1.00	64	16.00
5	1.25	65	16.25

Tax due on taxable pay from £100 to £23,700

Total taxable pay to date	Total tax due to date	Total taxable pay to date	Total tax due to date
£	£	£	£
100	25.00	6100	1525.00
200	50.00	6200	1550.00
300	75.00	6300	1575.00
400	100.00	6400	1600.00
500	125.00	6500	1625.00

Table B
(Lower rate relief)

Weekly pay

Week no.	Amount to substract
	£
1	1.93
2	3.85
3	5.77
4	7.70
5	9.62

Figure 21.1 Tax tables examples

Employee's surname *in CAPITALS* **SMITH**		First two forenames *SARAH LOUISE*	
National Insurance no. **TM 61 42 90 D**	**Date of birth** Day Month Year **21 07 72**	**Works no. etc**	**Date of leaving** Day Month Year

Tax Code	Amended code				
352L	Wk/Mth in which applied				

PAYE Income Tax

Wk No.	Pay in the week or month inc. SSP/SMP* 2	Total pay to date 3	Total free pay to date as shown by Table A 4	Total taxable pay to date 5	Total tax due to date as shown by taxable pay tables 6	Tax deducted or refunded in the week 7	For employer's use
	£	£	£	£	£	£	
1	132.00	132.00	67.68	64.32	14.07	14.07	
2	106.00	238.00	135.36	102.64	21.65	7.58	
3	129.00	367.00	203.04	163.96	34.98	13.33	
4							
5							
6							

*Statutory sick pay/statutory maternity pay

Figure 21.2   P11 deductions working sheet

Calculations are recorded on the deductions worksheet (P11). An example is shown in Figure 21.2, with some entries recorded. Except for columns 2 and 7, the figures accumulate over the year. The procedure for completing the form is as follows:

Column 2   The pay in the current week or month.

Column 3   Pay for the current week added to the total pay to date from the previous week. Hence for week 2:

	£
Pay in week 2	106.00
Total pay to date from week 1	132.00
Total pay to date for week 2	238.00

Column 4   Look up in Table A (pay adjustment tables) the free pay for the tax code and week number. From the example above, for code 352 the free pay in week 1 is £67.68. The tables contain a separate

page for each week of the tax year, with the free pay increasing each week. This spreads the tax free allowance evenly over the whole year. The tables (not shown) give the free pay for week 2 and code 352 as £135.36.

Column 5 total pay to date (column 3) minus free pay to date (column 4). Hence for week 2:

	£
Total pay to date for week 2	238.00
Free pay to date for week 2	135.36
Total taxable pay to date	102.64

Column 6 Tax due to date as shown by Table B. The calculation has to be made in several steps. For week 2, using the tables shown, the calculation is:

	£
Tax at 25% on £100	25.00
Tax at 25% on £2 (ignore the 64p)	0.50
Less lower rate relief for week 2	−3.85
Tax due to date for week 2	21.65

Column 7 The difference between the tax due to date for the current week, less tax already deducted as shown by the tax due to date for the previous week. For week 2:

	£
Tax due to date for week 2	21.65
Less tax already deducted	
(column 6 for week 1)	−14.07
Tax to deduct for week 2	7.58

Having calculated and made the necessary deductions, the money needs to be forwarded to the Inland Revenue on a regular basis.

Corporation Tax

If the business is run as a limited company, the profits are subject to corporation tax rather than income tax. Any money paid to the owners or directors of the business is subject to income tax. The decision to incorporate is complex and professional guidance based on individual circumstances is essential.

National Insurance Contributions

As with income tax, the business owner will be concerned with contributions for themselves and any employees.

Class 1 contributions are payable on employees' earnings, if they exceed a weekly minimum level. A figure for the employee's contribution has to be deducted from the pay in a similar way to the PAYE income tax deduction. The employer also contributes a percentage of the weekly earnings, thus increasing the cost of employing staff. These figures are recorded on the P11 form used for PAYE calculations.

Self employed people are liable to pay a Class 2 flat rate, unless their earnings are less than a very low threshold figure. In addition, Class 4 contributions, which are calculated as a percentage of profits, are also payable.

Value Added Tax (VAT)

VAT registration

A business must register for VAT if its sales of relevant goods and services during a year exceed, or are expected to exceed, a threshold figure. This is likely to include all but small stables businesses. Once registered, VAT has to be charged on all standard rated sales, and the money thus collected paid over to the Customs and Excise on a regular basis. To partly compensate, VAT paid on business expenses can be reclaimed.

Becoming VAT registered can have quite an effect on a business. Say a small livery yard has turnover below the registration threshold, and is charging £60 a week for full livery. If it expands and becomes VAT registered, the livery charge would have to increase to £60 + £10.50 VAT (at 17.5%), which is not likely to be popular with the livery owners. The alternative is to keep the charge at £60, in which case the business owner will only keep £51.07, £8.93 being VAT collected for the government.

VAT groupings

Not all goods and services are subject to VAT. They are classed into different groupings, with VAT only payable on those that are standard rated. Other items are classed as either zero rated, or exempt. Most sales from horse businesses are standard rated. Exceptions may be DIY livery (exempt) and grass livery (zero rated) if the service is merely for the provision of a stable or grazing. Livestock feed is zero rated. Examples of exempt supplies are insurance, wages and rent.

VAT records

Accurate records must be kept for VAT purposes, with documents retained for six years. All invoices must quote the VAT registration number of the business. The easiest way to keep the records is by incorporating them into the cash analysis book, as described in chapter 3. This option is only available to businesses that qualify for the cash accounting scheme by having an annual turnover of less than the prevailing limit.

Larger businesses have to keep records based on tax point dates, which are usually the same as the invoice date. This involves recording invoices as they are received or issued, and completing the VAT return from this data. VAT returns have to be completed and returned, with any tax collected during the period, usually every three months. Severe penalties can be applied by the Customs and Excise if returns are completed incorrectly or late. As with income tax, it is only genuine business expenses on which repayment of input tax can be claimed.

In addition to these records, a VAT account has to be kept, which summarises how the VAT return entries have been calculated.

Second-hand horses and ponies

Second-hand horses and ponies are subject to a special VAT scheme. This enables a VAT registered trader to charge VAT only on the difference between the purchase and selling prices of a horse, rather than the full selling price. To qualify, there are certain record keeping, invoicing and accounting requirements laid down by Customs and Excise. The horse must also have been bought from a private person, or someone selling it under the second-hand horse scheme. It is potentially very significant for a yard involved in dealing. Sales must be documented on a special form, which can be obtained from the British Equestrian Trade Association, Wothersome Grange, Bramham, West Yorkshire LS23 6LY.

Inheritance Tax

Inheritance tax is charged on lifetime gifts and transfers on death. Outright gifts to individuals are exempt from tax at the time of the gift, but if the donor dies within seven years of making the gift, tax will be payable. The value of an individual's estate, above a certain amount, is also taxed at the time of death.

Certain gifts are exempt from tax completely, including transfers between husband and wife, and small gifts to others.

An amount of relief may be available on the transfer of agricultural land and business property, during lifetime or on death. Any remaining tax then due can be paid over a period of ten years free of interest. These measures are intended to preserve the assets of family businesses on the death of the owner. A considerable tax liability can still remain, however, which can be reduced significantly by early planning for succession. This may include the passing down of assets to the next generation over a number of years during life, and taking full advantage of the tax free portion of the estate on the death of the first partner in a marriage.

Example

For example, a husband and wife own an estate worth £500,000, and the owners have four children.

Situation 1 – no tax planning

The wife inherits the full value of the estate on the death of her husband. When she dies, the tax liability is:

	£
Value of the estate	500,000
Slice of transfer free of tax (say)	200,000
Taxable transfer	300,000
Tax at 40%	120,000

Situation 2 – planning for succession

Permissible exempt gifts to children are £6,000 total per year, and are given for 10 years, before the death of the husband. Hence total lifetime gifts are £60,000. On the death of the husband, £200,000 is passed down to the children, and the remainder of the estate to the wife. The value of the estate on the death of the wife is therefore:

	£
Value of the estate	500,000
Less lifetime gifts	–60,000
Less transfer to children on death of husband	–200,000
Value of wife's estate on death	240,000
Slice of transfer free of tax	200,000
Taxable transfer on death of wife	40,000
Tax at 40%	16,000

In addition to taking full advantage of the available exemptions, life assurance policies can be taken out to contribute towards an expected tax liability on death.

Capital Gains Tax

Capital gains tax is a tax on the capital gains of individuals: gains by companies are charged to corporation tax. The tax is only charged when the gain is realised through sale of the asset. Any gain is calculated as the sale price less the acquisition value, less an allowance for inflation. The gain is then taxed at the rate of income tax that would apply if it was the top slice of income received by the individual. A small amount of capital gains can be realised, without any liability to tax, during each tax year. Any losses realised during the year can be offset against the gains.

Certain reliefs from capital gains tax are available on retirement. Principal private residences are exempt from tax. Tax on gains resulting from the sale of business assets can be deferred if the proceeds are spent on new assets, such as a qualifying new business, which are liable to the tax. The new assets must be acquired within set time limits before and after the sale of the original business.

Uniform Business Rates

This is a charge on business premises, which has had a major impact on a number of equine establishments. The rateable value of premises is based on a typical rent that could be obtained if they were let. A revaluation takes place every five years. Appeals against the valuation can be made to the local Valuation Agency office. To work out the rates payable in a year, the rateable value is multiplied by the current uniform business rate, set by central government.

Answers to Exercises

Chapter 3

(1) See cash analysis sheets (Figures 1 and 2).

(2) (a) VAT due on sales and other outputs   £3,852.36
    (b) VAT reclaimed on purchases and other inputs   £601.43
    (c) Net VAT to be paid to Customs and Excise   £3,250.93
    (d) Total value of sales and other outputs   £22,014
    (e) Total value of purchases and other inputs   £8,820

Date	Detail	Amount	Riding lessons	Livery fees	Sundry income	VAT on sales	Value of sales
01/06	Brought forward	17,084.02	11,895.74	3,009.60	247.00	2,651.67	15,152.34
03/06	B. Black – livery	280.00		226.30	12.00	41.70	238.30
06/06	Lessons wc 1/6	1,730.00	1,472.35			257.65	1,472.35
08/06	M. Smith – livery	164.00		124.58	15.00	24.42	139.58
13/06	Lessons wc 8/6	1,776.00	1,511.49			264.51	1,511.49
20/06	Lessons wc 15/6	1,812.00	1,542.13			269.87	1,542.13
23/06	M. Blenkinsop – livery	319.00		271.49		47.51	271.49
25/06	H. Jump – livery	86.00		73.20		12.80	73.20
27/06	Lessons wc 22/6	1,895.00	1,612.77			282.23	1,612.77
	Total for June	8,062.00	6,138.74	695.57	27.00	1,200.69	6,861.31
	Cum. total Apr–Jun	25,866.02	18,034.48	3,705.17	274.00	3,852.36	22,013.65

Figure 1   Oxhill Stables – cash analysis book – receipts

Date	Detail	Ch.	Amount	Feed, hay, straw	Vet. and med., farrier	Wages	Rent, rates property	Vehicle and power exps	Office and admin exps	Loan repayment	Private drawings	VAT on inputs	VAT to C&E	Value of inputs
01/06	Brought forward		17,702.36	2,280.00	505.00	4,660.00	4,104.00	174.00	620.00	1,000.00	1,300.00	525.36	2,534.00	7,397.00
12/06	District Council	129	286.00				286.00							
19/06	Compton Times ad.	130	99.88						85.00			14.88		85.00
26/06	Wages	131	2,300.00			2,300.00								
26/06	Private drawings	132	580.00								580.00			
30/06	Feed Supplies	133	520.00	520.00										520.00
30/06	Jab & Hope (Vets)	134	263.91		224.60							39.31		224.60
30/06	J. Straw – bedding	135	400.00	400.00										400.00
30/06	Spanner & Bodgit	136	146.88					125.00				21.88		125.00
30/6	Bank Charges		68.50						68.50					68.50
	Total for June		4,665.17	920.00	224.60	2,300.00	286.00	125.00	153.50	0.00	580.00	76.07	0.00	1,423.10
	Cum. total Apr–June		22,367.53	3,200.00	729.60	6,960.00	4,390.00	299.00	773.50	1,000.00	1,880.00	601.43	2,534.00	8,820.10

Figure 2 Oxhill Stables – cash analysis book – payments

Chapter 4

(1) Balance Sheet on 31 October 199_

	£	£
Fixed assets		
Premises	250,000	
Vehicles	14,000	
Brood mares	8,000	
		272,000
Current assets		
Young horses	9,000	
Debtors	500	
Cash	50	
	9,550	
Current liabilities		
Bank overdraft	5,000	
Trade creditors	1,200	
	6,200	
Net current assets		**3,350**
Long-term liabilities		
Mortgage		50,000
Net capital		**225,350**
Financed by:		
Opening net capital		218,350
Add: net profit for the year		17,000
		235,350
Subtract: private drawings		(10,000)
		225,350

(2) Trading profit and loss account for the year ending 31 October 199_

	£	£
Sales		80,000
Less cost of sales		
Opening stock	7,000	
Direct costs	20,000	
	27,000	
Less closing stock	(9,000)	
		18,000
Gross profit		**62,000**
Overhead expenses		45,000
Net profit		**17,000**

Chapter 8

(1) Potential of existing business
     Gross margins

	£
Full livery horses	
Sales	3,000
Variable costs	800
Gross margin per horse	2,200

	£
DIY livery horses	
Sales	1,000
Variable costs	200
Gross margin per horse	800

	£
Dealing horses	
Sales	3,200
Variable costs	
Purchase	1,800
Direct costs	250
Gross margin per horse	1,150

System budget – existing system

Gross margins	£	£
7 Full liveries @	2,200	15,400
5 DIY liveries @	800	4,000
6 Dealing horses @	1,150	6,900
Total gross margin		26,300

Overhead expenses	
Labour	9,000
Rates	1,800
Other	8,000
Total overhead expenses	18,800

Net profit	**7,500**

(2) Potential after expansion
     Gross margins

	£
Full livery horses	
Sales	3,250
Variable costs	800
Gross margin per horse	2,450

	£
DIY livery horses	
Sales	1,100
Variable costs	200
Gross margin per horse	900

Dealing horses
Unchanged

Breaking and schooling	£
Sales	540
Variable costs	100
Gross margin per horse	440

System budget – after expansion

Gross margins	£	£
12 Full liveries @	2,450	29,400
8 DIY liveries @	900	7,200
6 Dealing horses @	1,150	6,900
12 Breaking and schooling @	440	5,280
Total gross margin		48,780
Overhead expenses		
Labour		15,000
Rates		3,800
Other		15,000
Total overhead expenses		33,800
Net profit		**14,980**

Chapter 9

(1) Profit forecast for the year commencing 1 Jan 199_

	£	£
Sales		
Full livery fees	30,875	
DIY livery fees	7,150	
Horses	19,200	
		57,225
Less cost of sales		
Opening stock	3,000	
Horses	10,800	
Cost of sales	10,400	
	24,200	
Less closing stock	(3,000)	
		21,200
Gross profit		36,025
Overheads (fixed costs)		
Labour		12,000
Rates		3,800
Building depreciation		2,000
Interest on loan		4,000
Other		11,000
		32,800
Net profit		**3,225**

Explanation of some figures:

Full livery fees	7 horses @ £3,250	22,750
	5 horses @ £1,625	8,125
		30,875
Horse sales	6 horses @ £3,200	19,200

Cost of sales:

Full liveries	7 horses @ £800	5,600
	5 horses @ £400	2,000
DIY liveries	5 horses @ £200	1,000
	3 horses @ £100	300
Dealing	6 horses @ £250	1,500
		10,400

Labour £9,000, plus extra £3,000

Chapter 10

(1) Cashflow forecast for Jan–June

	Jan	Feb	Mar	Apr	May	June
Receipts						
Lessons	1,200	900	1,100	1,400	1,400	1,300
VAT on outputs	210	158	193	245	245	228
Total	1,410	1,058	1,293	1,645	1,645	1,528
Payments						
Horses and tack			4000			
Feed, bedding	400	400	400	400	200	200
Labour	400	400	400	500	500	500
Rates				1,000		
Other	300	300	300	300	300	300
Interest @ 10%	0	0	0	22	27	22
VAT on inputs	53	53	53	53	53	53
VAT to C&E			403			560
Total	1,153	1,153	5,556	2,275	1,080	1,635
Net cash flow	257	−95	−4,263	−630	565	−107
Opening bank	1,500	1,757	1,662	−2,601	−3,231	−2,666
Closing bank	1,757	1,662	−2,601	−3,231	−2,666	−2,773

(2) An overdraft limit of £3,500 would be appropriate, to cover the forecast balance of −£3,231 in April.

Chapter 11

(1) Reconciliation of profit and cash flow forecasts for the year commencing 1/4/95

	£
Net profit	22,918
+ depreciation	2,300
+ loans taken out	0
+ decrease in stocks	3,033
– loan repayments	(4,000)
– personal drawings and tax	(9,000)
– capital investments	0
= **Net cash flow for the year**	**15,251**

From cashflow forecasts

	£
Opening bank balance	(20,560)
Closing bank balance	(5,309)
Net cash flow	**15,251**

Projected balance sheet on 31/3/96

Fixed assets	£	£
Buildings		18,400
Vehicles		4,500
School horses and ponies		20,333
Tack and equipment		4,500
		47,733
Current assets		
Bank balance	0	
Current liabilities		
Bank overdraft	5,309	
Net current assets		(5,309)
Long-term liability		
Loan		12,000
Net capital		**30,424**

Chapter 13

(1) Replace four DIY liveries with four more school horses.

Extra income	£	£
School horses 4 @ £4,400		17,600
Total gains		**17,600**
Income lost		
DIY liveries 4 @ £900	3,600	
Extra costs		
School horse variable 4 @ £1,200	4,800	
Replacement cost (£1,800–£1,000)		

$$\frac{\text{Replacement cost (£1,800–£1,000)}}{4 \text{ years}}$$

	£	£
= 4 horses @ £200	800	
Interest £7,200 @ 12%	864	
Extra labour	3,000	
		9,464
Total losses		**13,064**
Extra profit		**4,536**

(2) Own haymaking machinery instead of using contractor

Costs saved

	£
Contractor's charge 10 ha @ £120	1,200

Extra costs

Machinery depreciation (£5,000–£1,000)

	£
4 years	1,000
Spares and repairs for machinery	250
Tractor running costs for hay making	200
Interest on capital £5,000 @ 10%	500
	1,950
Loss	**(750)**

The business is £750 better off by using the services of the contractor.

Chapter 14

Sensitivity analysis

1(b) Sensitivity analysis of school ponies' gross margin
Lesson price +/− £1/hour (excluding VAT), gross margin +/− £460
(£1/hour × 10 hours/week × 46 weeks = £460)

Teaching hours +/− 1 hour/week,
gross margin +/− £509
(1 hour × £11.06 (ex. VAT) × 46 weeks = £509)

1(c) Sensitivity analysis of livery horses' gross margin
Livery fee +/− £5/week (excluding VAT), gross margin +/− £225
(£5/week × 45 weeks/year = £225)
Facility uptake +/− 1 week/year, gross margin +/− £510
(1 week × £63.83 (ex. VAT) = £63.83)

Break even analysis

(1) The business will break even with just over 14 horses (Figure 3). Profit with 20 horses is £20,000.

(2) Break even point is 11 horses. Profit with 20 horses is £40,000.

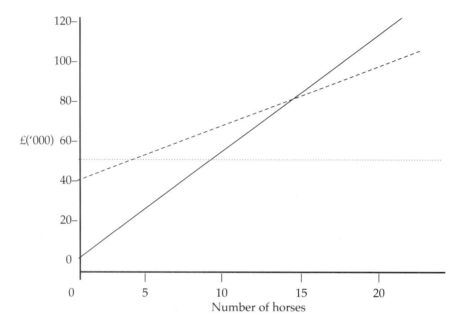

Figure 3   Break even analysis

Chapter 15

1(a) Pay back period

		£
Investment		27,000
Cumulative net cash flow		
Year	1	5,000
	2	16,000
	3	27,000
	4	38,000

Pay back period (years)   3.0
Both options achieve a pay back in around three years, number two being slightly quicker.

1(b) Annual rate of return

Year	Net cash flow £	Net profit £
1	5,000	3,500
2	11,000	9,500
3	11,000	9,500
4	11,000	9,500
5	11,000	9,500
		41,500
Average annual net profit		8,300

Annual rate of return = $\dfrac{£8,300 \times 100}{£27,000}$

= 30.7%

Like the livery option, this yields a high rate of return, but even better.

1(c) Net present value (NPV)

Year	Net cash flow £	Discount factor	NPV £
0	(27,000)	1.000	(27,000)
1	5,000	0.909	4,545
2	11,000	0.826	9,091
3	11,000	0.751	8,264
4	11,000	0.683	7,513
5	11,000	0.621	6,830
			9,243

Both projects give a positive NPV at 10% discount rate, with the highest figure produced by the school horses option.

1(d) Internal rate of return (IRR)
NPV using a discount rate of 20%

Year	Net cash flow £	Discount factor	NPV £
0	(27,000)	1.000	(27,000)
1	5,000	0.833	4,167
2	11,000	0.694	7,639
3	11,000	0.579	6,366
4	11,000	0.482	5,305
5	11,000	0.402	4,421
			898

If the NPV values using the discount rates of 10% and 20% are plotted on a graph, it can be seen that the IRR is approximately 21.1%. This is higher than that achieved by the livery option.

(2) Each of the four techniques favours using the new stables for school horses. Both of the options appear to be worthwhile investments.

Chapter 17

1(a) Business A – sources and applications of funds statement for the year ending 31 March 199_

Sources of funds	£	Applications of funds	£
Net profit	18,000	Private drawings	11,000
Depreciation	5,000	Tax	3,000
		Capital investment	12,000
		Increase in debtors	2,000
		Increase in stocks	3,000
	23,000		31,000
Decrease in bank balance			**(8,000)**

1(b) **Business B – sources and applications of funds statement for the year ending 31 March 199_**

Sources of funds	£	Applications of funds	£
Net profit	6,000	Private drawings	7,000
Depreciation	5,000	Increase in debtors	20
Decrease in stocks	3,000	Capital investment	2,500
Increase in creditors	2,000		
	16,000		9,520
Increase in bank balance			**6,480**

Comments

Business A

The net profit more than covers the private drawings and tax, with £4,000 surplus. The profitability of the business is adequate. The bank balance has declined because of increased stocks and capital investments, both of which should lead to greater profits in the future. The business appears to be in a sound position.

Business B

Here the business has made a cash surplus, but for unhealthy reasons. Stocks have decreased and creditors increased. Investment has been less than the depreciation allowance. This suggests that the assets of the business are being run down, which will affect its future profitability. Most important, the private drawings are greater than the profit, which is at a low level and needs to be increased.

(2) **Sources and applications of funds statement for Oxhill Stables for the year ending 31 March 1996**

Sources of funds	£	Applications of funds	£
Net profit	25,261	Increase in debtors	180
Depreciation	2,300	Loan repayment	4,000
Decrease in stocks	2,570	Private and tax	8,340
Increase in creditors	35		
	30,166		12,520
Increase in bank balance			**17,646**

Closing bank balance	(1,849)
Opening bank balance	(19,495)
	17,646

Sources of figures

Net profit and depreciation – from the TP&L account.
Decrease in stocks – difference between closing and opening stock in the TP&L account.
Increase in creditors – difference between closing and opening creditors on the balance sheets.
Loan repayment – from loans on the balance sheets.
Private and tax – from the 'Financed by' section of the balance sheet.

Chapter 18

(1) The most significant trends are the declines in net capital, net current assets and bank balance, all of which are undesirable.

Assets have been maintained, and there must have been some investment in a new vehicle. This was perhaps unwise when the money was not available, and is likely to have caused the deterioration in net current assets and bank balance. Profit was insufficient to cover the private drawings and tax. These need to be reduced, or preferably profits increased, in the future.

(2) Ratio calculations:

	30 Sept 96	1 Oct 95
Owner equity %	£172,975	£176,450
	£225,175	£223,195
	= 77%	= 79%

These figures are borderline, and the trend needs to show improvement rather than a continued decline.

Capital gearing	£40,000	£40,000
	£172,975	£176,450
	= 23%	= 23%

Current ratio	£11,675	£11,195
	£12,200	£6,745
	= 96%	= 166%

Liquidity ratio	£375	£745
	£12,200	£6,745
	= 3%	= 11%

The short-term cash availability is poor and reducing the overdraft should be a priority.

Return on capital employed
$$\frac{£9,400}{£212,975}$$
$$= 4\%$$

This represents a low rate of return that could be bettered (with much less risk) by depositing the money with a bank.

Chapter 19

Year ending 30 September	1996	1995
(1) Gross profit %	$\frac{£49,860}{£124,000}$	$\frac{£48,730}{£117,150}$
	= 40%	= 42%
Net profit %	$\frac{£13,780}{£124,000}$	$\frac{£16,530}{£117,150}$
	= 11%	= 14%

Despite increased sales, profitability has fallen. This appears to be due to two factors:

❑   a reduced mark-up on sales leading to lower gross profit %;
❑   an increase in overheads.

The business needs to try and raise prices and control overheads.

(2) Stock turnover	$\frac{£74,140}{£7,250}$	$\frac{£68,420}{£6,150}$
	= 10.2	= 11.1 times
or	36	33 days

More careful stock control is needed to increase the turnover.

(3) Credit given	$\frac{£1,300 \times 365}{£124,000}$	$\frac{£900 \times 365}{£117,150}$
	= 4	= 3 days
Credit taken	$\frac{£3,200 \times 365}{£75,640}$	$\frac{£3,500 \times 365}{£69,120}$
	= 15	= 18 days

There is no problem with debtors. It is worth investigating whether full use is being made of credit offered by suppliers, as 15 days is not a long period.

(4) Interest cover	$\frac{£15,780}{£2,000}$	$\frac{£18,030}{£1,500}$
	= 7.9	= 12.0 times

The business is having no problems with covering its interest charges, although these are increasing and need to be controlled.

General comments

The health of the business is getting worse, mainly because it did not manage to make enough profit in 1995/6. It needs to increase its profit in the next year, by a combination of:

❑ raising prices
❑ increasing sales
❑ controlling costs (of stock and overheads)
❑ better stock control.

Chapter 20

(1) School horses	Total £	Per horse £
Sales		
Lessons	49,680	4,140
Variable costs		
Feed	3,120	260
Hay	3,360	280
Bedding	720	60
Veterinary and medicines	600	50
Farrier	720	60
Grassland expenses	180	15
Replacement cost*	300	25
	9,000	750
Gross margin	**40,680**	**3,390**
*Replacement cost		
Opening stock	10,200	
Closing stock	(10,800)	
Horse purchased	1,500	
Horse sold	(600)	
	300	25

Livery horses	Total £	Per horse £
Sales		
Livery fees	24,960	3,120
Variable costs		
Feed	1,880	235
Hay	2,240	280
Bedding	480	60
Grassland expenses	120	15
	4,720	590
Gross margin	**20,240**	**2,530**

(2) Lower sales through fewer lessons or lower prices; higher variable costs such as feed and bedding.

(3) Different overhead expenses – the school is likely to have extra costs for:

- ❑ interest charges – because the horses are owned
- ❑ labour
- ❑ buildings
- ❑ general administration and insurances.

Index